# IMPROBABLE JOY

## A 3-TIME CANCER SURVIVOR'S JOURNEY TO OVERCOMING FEAR AND PAIN

KIPP HARRIS

Difference Press

Washington, DC, USA

Copyright © Kipp Harris, 2022

All rights reserved. No part of this book may be reproduced in any form without permission in writing from the author. Reviewers may quote brief passages in reviews.

Published 2022

DISCLAIMER

No part of this publication may be reproduced or transmitted in any form or by any means, mechanical or electronic, including photocopying or recording, or by any information storage and retrieval system, or transmitted by email without permission in writing from the author.

Neither the author nor the publisher assumes any responsibility for errors, omissions, or contrary interpretations of the subject matter herein. Any perceived slight of any individual or organization is purely unintentional.

Brand and product names are trademarks or registered trademarks of their respective owners.

Cover Design: Jennifer Stimson

Editing: Cory Hott

Author Photo Credit: Stacy Kennedy, StacyKennedy.com

# CONTENTS

*Foreword* — vii
*Introduction: My Story* — ix

1. Life Isn't Fair — 1
2. Stop Fighting Cancer — 5
3. Share Your Story and Your Journey — 13
4. Find a Way to Create Your Own Epiphany — 17
5. Beginning the Chemotherapy Journey — 31
6. Embracing the Chemotherapy Journey — 49
7. Finding Joy in the Chemotherapy Journey — 67
8. Change Your Life Even after Chemo — 83

*Conclusion: Pain and Joy Exist Simultaneously* — 111
*Acknowledgments* — 119
*About the Author* — 123

*From the time I was a young boy, the foundation of life and all that matters has been love. This understanding of what's truly important is not innate, but rather, it's something that has to be learned. I consider myself lucky to have been born into love!*

*While no family is perfect. and I would imagine that every parent can recognize "mistakes" made along the way, I believe that every part of who I am today has been manifested through all the experiences of my life. Undoing that which some consider "bad" would, inevitably, change who I am in this moment. And I like who I am today and owe that primarily to two people: my parents!*

*From an early age, I was taught not to quit. If I started something and realized I didn't like it, I had to finish and honor the commitment I made. Engrained in my DNA are the words, "If you tell the truth, you can remember what you say." So much of who I am today was fertilized at a very young age and nurtured with consistent love. For this, my gratitude again extends to two people: my parents!*

*I believe this book only exists today because I was taught by them to forge on and never give up. Additionally, in their own way, they helped me find the strength to see something good in even the most difficult moments. Love holds my family together. And this book is written with love for my parents, Jack and Billiette.*

# FOREWORD

It was our fortieth wedding anniversary trip. My husband and I had already been to Branson, Missouri, for a few days, and now we were in the car driving to Mount Rushmore, where we would spend another day or two. My cell phone rang, and I noticed it was our son Kipp calling. I answered the phone and could hear in Kipp's voice that this was not a social call to see how we were enjoying our trip. Kipp told me that he was in the hospital in California where he lived and was going to have his appendix removed in the morning. "You don't have to come; I'll be fine," is what he said to me. Of course, moms always know when they are needed so we changed our travel plans and went home to North Dakota instead of visiting Mount Rushmore. Once we arrived at home, I packed a different suitcase, made flight reservations, and flew to California to be with our son.

Surgery diagnosis was much more than we had expected. It was not a simple appendectomy but a rare cancer of the appendix. In that moment, I recalled a daily devotional that a friend had shared with me years earlier when we first found out that our son, Kipp is gay. "I shall try to remember dear Lord that you do not send trouble our way, but rather the strength to endure it." God was with us when we went through the trials of our son's coming out process, and I knew that He would be with us now as we would go through another difficult time in our life.

In the next three years, our family would be involved with Kipp enduring three major cancer surgeries, plus intense chemotherapy with each surgery. This was not an easy time for us. Kipp, however, found a way to get through his journey by "looking for the *joy*." I have also had cancer, but I did not experience the joy like Kipp. (Maybe my mindset was not looking hard enough?) That is my loss because I know for sure that Kipp did find joy.

The stories in this book are about real people. The flashbacks are honest, funny, and inspiring. They are moments where Kipp recalls finding joy during his cancer journey. I think he shares these brief times with us so that we can be more aware of our moments. We *can* make a difference, and sometimes we don't even know that we do.

No one wants trouble in their life, but when it comes, maybe it's a test of our faith, or perhaps we can acquire a new strength from it? If love is found in the heart of our trials, I have faith that we can overcome anything.

Our family is a circle of love and strength. Every crisis faced makes our circle stronger and every joy shared adds more love. In this book, "joy" is "love smiling."

I love you, Kipp

— MOM

# INTRODUCTION: MY STORY

When diagnosed with cancer in September 2004, my thoughts spiraled when I learned that six months of chemotherapy would be the ultimate treatment plan, and the side effects could possibly prevent me from working. I worried that all my years of climbing the corporate ladder would be thrown away when people saw me struggle through the rigors of chemotherapy. In corporate America, the weak get left behind. Hard work means long hours and stepping up to the plate even when nobody asks. Having climbed the corporate ladder from trainer to sales, to regional manager, I was responsible for eleven states, Guam and Saipan, overseeing three regional offices on the west coast for a company based on the east coast of the United States. I took pride in my ability to be seen as a leader and had worked hard to gain the respect of my colleagues. If I knew then what I know now, I would not have wasted so much energy on things I can't control.

In June 2004, I decided to train for a marathon. I'd always been in relatively good shape, but knowing that I would be running the longest distance of my life in six months, I began a rigorous training schedule. I ran daily, and while things were mostly going well, I noticed side aches during some of my nightly runs. After a couple of months, the pain sustained and didn't go away quickly, so I made an appointment to see my primary care physician. Of course, by the time I got in to see her, the pain had receded, and she dismissed it as muscular pain due to my increased training activities. I agreed with her and moved on – but the pain came back. Knowing that it was just muscular, I persisted, and eventually the pain subsided, so I continued training.

In September 2004, I decided to take the afternoon off from work and head north to China Camp State Park in Marin County, California, where I had often done mountain biking. It was a gorgeous midweek day, and the trail was quiet which made for perfect riding conditions. As I trekked up the singletrack trails winding back and forth to reach the top, my mind reflected on life, and I became excited anticipating the arrival of my boyfriend that evening. I was, at the time, in a long-distance relationship where he lived on the east coast and I on the west coast. It had been several weeks since we'd seen each other, and I was even more excited when I found a new trailhead that I had never seen before this day. I hit that trail and ventured down the mountain again imagining that Bernie would enjoy this tomorrow with me, as our plans were to ride together the next day.

As I moved toward the base of the trail, my side ached more painfully than it ever had. With marathon training, I was getting used to the minor side aches, but this was out of control. When I finally reached my car, the pain was so bad I had to have someone nearby lift my bike to the top of my car. Driving home, I thought about seeking medical attention but again dismissed it as muscular pain. When I picked Bernie up at the airport, he could see I was in excruciating pain, and, of course, I ended up in the emergency room later that night. My diagnosis was initially an atypical presentation of appendicitis. However, the surgery revealed what appeared to be cancer on my appendix, so the surgeon removed the tumors along with portions of both my small and large intestines. In the years to follow, I recognized that symptoms are not meant to be ignored the way I did.

It was Labor Day weekend when I had my emergency surgery, so the pathology that confirmed my cancer diagnosis was not learned until almost a week later. In that waiting period, my parents had come from North Dakota to California and were now living with me as I embarked on the journey to figure out what came next.

I really believe physicians are much like commodities to lay people who don't understand the complexities of the human body. They have the information I need, but it is my job to decide what happens. I'm a big advocate for patients taking control of their situation, and so I interviewed three different oncologists to figure out what the best treatment for me would be. Ultimately, I chose Martha Tracy, an oncologist in Berkeley who my parents did not really like. She was clinical – and I liked that aspect of her. I had my parents, friends, and family for hugs and love; what I needed from my physician was a thorough understanding and concrete plan to kick cancer's butt. Over the years, and as I will share in this book, that approach served me well. In the years to follow, I received two more diagnoses of the same recurrence of appendiceal cancer. I was always told the odds of survival were fifty-fifty, and that proved true as I have met three other people with the same type of cancer – two are gone, and two of us are still here.

This feels like the right place to acknowledge and recognize someone of great importance in my life. She was the first person I knew who had cancer. Vi Gartner was the bookkeeper at my parent's business in Kenmare, North Dakota. As a kid, I worked at "the shop" every summer and would spend many of my coffee breaks sitting in Vi's office chatting with her. Those moments connecting with Vi over a break in her office are, to this day, some of my most cherished memories. I think having conversations with her when I was still a high school student taught me early on the value of relationships with other people. Today, connection is one of the foundations of my life and I wonder if it didn't start with Vi.

One hot summer day, I walked into Vi's office to take my break, and the smell of my great grandma Elsie's perfume emanated strongly. As a child, I would go stay with my grandma in Williston, North Dakota, where she ran the local bus depot. She lived in an apartment in the back of the building, and the entire apartment always smelled like "Grandma Elsie." It was a distinct smell, and I guess it stuck with me over the years. Walking into Vi's office that day, I smelled that same odor and asked her, "Did you get new perfume?" She laughed and said, "Kipp, I just sprayed fly spray in my office." We both laughed, and it became clear after so many years had passed that my great grandma did not wear a stinky perfume – she had a huge fly problem at the bus depot.

I remember staying at Vi's house one weekend when my parents had to go out of town. She lived in an old two-story house by herself and even today, those memories stick with me. Connecting with Vi over a break while working was one thing, but spending a weekend with her was quite another. Of course, I never told her this, but I always admired her for being so independent. Her husband had passed away at a young age and she continued living in the big old house on the hill in Kenmare. As a kid, I saw her as an example of strength and independence. In ways she never knew, I really idolized her and loved her. On March 23, 1988, I was home from college, and I went to the hospital in the morning to visit Vi. Her cancer had progressed, and she died later that day. I still remember walking up to her bedside and touching her hand to say hello. She couldn't speak, but as she looked into my eyes and acknowledged my presence, I said, "How are you doing?" The stupidity of that question at that moment right before her death still haunts me. But in the end, I know she loved me, and I have no doubt she was and is aware of my deep love and respect for her – even though neither of us said it.

Vi was the first person I ever knew who died from cancer, and even in that moment at the hospital when I asked such a stupid question, I still remember it as one of the most beautiful moments of my life. I know she was in pain, but even then, I found something joyful in being there with her. I didn't know it at the time, but this would be a sort of precursor to how I would handle my own cancer journey nearly twenty years later.

I do understand the fear and anger associated with an initial cancer diagnosis. Anger, for me, was a short-lived emotion; I'm lucky to have been able to move past it as quickly as I did. That said, I know cancer is a scary thing, and it conjures up all kinds of fear and emotion. How will my life change? Will I be able to keep working? Will I be able to care for my kids? Will I lose my hair? Will I be sick – or too weak to do anything? All these questions are valid and understandable, and I don't want to invalidate any of these feelings. My goal, however, is to help you not simply move past those feelings but work inside them. By this, I mean recognize and understand that nothing in life is easy. But if you focus only on the hardship, I believe you will miss out on seeing some really amazing things as you move through this experience.

I have learned a lot while undergoing surgery and chemotherapy thrice, most of which I'll share with you in this book. Acknowledging that life isn't fair is perhaps one of the first hurdles to overcome for many. Confronting and disposing of the "why me" mentality may be the first step in moving through cancer in a positive and productive way. I was lucky and will share my experience in getting there quite quickly. Creating space for intention is perhaps the most important thing I learned, and so I will spend a bit of time sharing my story about how I made this happen for me.

And while it might seem at odds with everything we know about cancer, I will encourage people to stop fighting cancer and instead embrace the journey and the experience. By moving away from the fight, I believe there are things awaiting you that otherwise can't be seen in the midst of battle. I further believe – and it may seem harsh to some – that this is the journey you are meant to have in life. Cancer and chemotherapy are part of your life experience, and selfishly taking that on by yourself doesn't serve anyone. Learning to share the experience with others by reaching out and asking for help will, in ways you can't yet see, benefit both you and the friends and family that walk with you. Once you learn and appreciate that your diagnosis impacts the lives of everyone around you, it will be time to create intention. This will be the key to finding joy as you experience fear and pain as you forge ahead. It is only by finding intentionality that you will be able to manifest love, joy, and connection through what many perceive as the agony of chemotherapy. By embracing and accepting this as part of your life experience, it will be possible to move past the anger that many feel at the time of diagnosis. Once you stop being angry, new doors will open, and you will be able to see all the amazing things that are happening – even in those moments when you might be dealing with pain or fear.

Joy does exist amidst pain and in the pages that follow, I will relay countless stories of those moments where I found joy in really unexpected places. Even today, having been cancer free for many years, I continue to seek out joy in the moments of my life where things don't go exactly the way I want. In my speaking events, I continue to challenge people in every facet of their life to look for joy. I am keenly aware of how everyday life brings challenges that don't exist when undergoing treatment. Life gets busy and it may be challenging to look for the good. Today, I take every opportunity available to remind people that joy does exist in parallel to all the troubling things encountered in life. For this reason, I am always reminding people to look for it.

1

## LIFE ISN'T FAIR

Getting an initial cancer diagnosis can be jarring, and it certainly throws a wrench into any normalcy one might have had in their daily routine. Even when I tried to just forge ahead, the thoughts in the back of my mind found their way forward only to interrupt my day. I imagined losing my hair, losing weight, vomiting, and being so tired from chemotherapy that I would not be able to work. The endless barrage of fear and anxiety became overwhelming at times.

Coming to terms with my cancer diagnosis took several weeks, but eventually, I got there. In the beginning, I reached out to family members and close friends to let them know what was happening in my life. Those phone calls almost always went the same way: I told the story of my mountain biking and then ending up in the emergency room. I finished the story with the emergency surgery and, ultimately, the pathology report that revealed a rare form of cancer that required six months of chemotherapy starting as soon as possible. Nearly without exception, I got virtually the same response: "Kipp, I'm so sorry." Most went on to exclaim the unfairness of my diagnosis and wrapped up the conversation by assuring me I would be in their thoughts and prayers. All of these responses came from love. Every single person with whom I had a conversation cared for me and genuinely wished that I didn't have to go through the pain of cancer and chemotherapy. I really did feel loved.

Somewhere around 1999, I met J.L. while skiing in Aspen, Colorado, and we both found an immediate connection in each other. He's nearly thirty years older than me but the generation gap was easily bridged by our mutual interests. J.L. is an outspoken, intelligent, well-read individual who thrives on deep and interesting conversation. He and I hit it off during that first meeting. And while skiing, he had no problem speaking up to tell me what I was doing wrong. On that ski trip, I excelled and found a passion for downhill skiing that had previously never existed. While I always enjoyed it, I finally loved it. He taught me how to ski mogul runs and before long, I was bouncing across the bumps as if they were clouds. It took many more years after I met J.L. to get really good, but, eventually, I got there. We became great friends, and today, I consider him one of my best friends.

When I called J.L. to tell him the news of my cancer diagnosis, I probably shouldn't have expected the typical response. After telling J.L. about my diagnosis, he simply said, "Well, Kipp, nobody said life was fair. And nobody said it was easy." What? Excuse me. Wow. I still become emotional every time I think about this moment. No apology. No rant about how difficult it was going to be. Just the truth. And it was the truth. In that moment, for the first time during all that had happened, I felt something shift. I wasn't going to succumb to the typical "fighting" mentality that accompanied most cancer stories. I believe J.L.

provided me with a moment that would change the course of my treatment. I didn't really know it at the time, but as I will show in this book, J.L. was the "spark that lit the fire" to create intention.

Now that I had this awareness that life really isn't fair, I had to embark on a mission to find the best treatment plan for me. People often ask, "why me?' but rarely ask, "why not me?" In his own way, J.L. boldly reminded me that life isn't fair, and so now I had a choice: wallow or move forward. In my life, I have noticed that people often take the advice of one physician without question. It seems we put them on pedestals as if they are God-like and don't question their authority and opinion. I understand that a cancer diagnosis is scary and when someone gives us hope, reaching out and taking that open hand of authority is often the easiest thing to do. My advice is that every cancer patient should seek treatment and options from multiple physicians. I interviewed three oncologists and, in the end, decided to work with Martha Tracy, a short, stout, braless, long-haired, Birkenstock-wearing woman who lacked a real bedside manner but made up for it with pinpoint clarity on what clinical approach needed to be taken to combat the rare cancer I had. My parents did not like her as she tended to ignore them and was hyper-focused on me and my questions. She is exactly what I needed. My parents provided me with love, support, hugs, and care when I needed it. My oncologist provided a treatment plan to kill the cancer. I recommend this approach but recognize it doesn't work for everyone.

After I finally made a decision to work with Dr. Tracy, I met with her to finalize the treatment plan. I was diagnosed in September, and she wanted to get started right away. However, I had a trip to Spain planned for November, and I explained to her that I really didn't want to miss it. At that point, I believe I started complaining to her about how I was also going to miss my annual ski trip to Whistler, British Columbia. I remember so vividly sitting in the small clinic room having this conversation. I told her about this trip that I took every year with friends from around the world, and, in short, I was probably feeling sorry for myself. Being that clinical-minded physician, I remember her turning to look at me with a quick retort, "Why don't you just go to South America and ski when you're done with chemo?" Not only did she find a quick and simple solution to my "problem" about not being able to ski this winter because I would be undergoing chemotherapy, but she gave me a solution that also instilled hope for the future. She was telling me that it was all going to be okay, and I would be able to just ski this summer in South America instead of this winter in North America. While her bedside manner might seem cold to many, she clearly cared, and in her own way, provided more hope than I could have imagined in that moment.

Yes, life isn't fair. And why not me? Why not you? I have learned nobody really deserves to endure pain, but I also believe that if you can find a way to forge ahead, the lessons you learn along the way will be life-changing and far more impactful than any temporary pain that may exist during that same time period. Open yourself up to the possibility that this journey you are about to embark on has a purpose. It might seem crazy and maybe even unfair, but focusing on the inequity of it won't make it go away. You've got this – if you only open up to the idea that maybe there's a greater lesson to be learned. How you move forward and the experience you have is all determined by you – and only you.

2

## STOP FIGHTING CANCER

*"This systematic review and synthesis of qualitative evidence drew out the multidimensionality of cancer fear. Cancer fears emanated from a core view of cancer as an enemy, evoking fears about its proximity, the (lack of) strategies available to keep it at a distance, the personal and social implications of succumbing, and dying from cancer. The view of cancer as an enemy seems widely reinforced in society but may impede effective cancer control strategies and the adoption of preventive health behaviours. Future policies should focus on removing mixed messages in the public portrayal of cancer."*

— PSYCHO-ONCOLOGY RESEARCH FEAR OF CANCER

After getting my treatment plan in place with my oncologist, I felt as if I had a strategy to embark on the mission. Ultimately, I just wanted the cancer out of me, and I wanted to get on with life. Yes, I was saddened by all that I would lose out on – my ski trip with friends most notably – but Dr. Tracy reminded me that life and my perspective could be shifted in a moment. I could make a small change and still have a ski trip, even if it looked a little different than past years.

I have heard it many times from people both before and after my cancer diagnosis: "You have to fight cancer if you want to survive." Hearing this so much, it seemed like the path I was inevitably going to take. In my mind, the twelve-week treatment plan proposed was my fight, and I would endure and finish it no matter what the side effects might be. Being a strong person, I started from a position where there really was no other option. I had the plan in place and was determined to move through chemotherapy and continue working so as not to be seen by anyone as weak.

When I started chemo the first time, reality hit me hard as I was unable to tolerate the drugs, and it became clear I would not be able to continue life and work as usual. Ultimately, I had to stop eating and was fed through a tube in my chest every night. Putting food into my stomach caused such unbearable pain that the only solution was to stop eating. This meant nutrition now went to my bloodstream directly, and I was constantly hungry having an empty stomach. I felt weak, especially having picked up some books about a rockstar chemo patient who thrived through chemo without any bumps in the road. I'd read a book by a famous athlete who never missed a thing going through chemotherapy. For the first time, I felt weak. Even in the midst of my waning positive mindset, I was able to forge ahead, and this had much to do with the intention I had created.

In the years that followed my initial cancer diagnosis, I learned a lot about fighting and what that mental position does to not only our bodies but our minds. There is clear and substantial research that supports the idea that when you fight against something (in this case, cancer), your mind is already absorbing the idea that you might lose. If this is just a win/ lose battle, then odds are not great, in my opinion. Given this, I believe you should move forward and accept cancer, chemotherapy, and whatever surgery or radiation might be required as part of the journey you are meant to have in life.

If you stop "fighting" cancer, that doesn't mean you have to give up the quest to rid it from your body. It just means that you acknowledge it and choose to focus on the entirety of your life in the moment – not just the cancer. Preoccupying your thoughts and actions with one sole purpose – fighting cancer – you will, without a doubt, miss out on things happening around you. I truly believe and have stories to prove that when you accept what is, you open the doors and windows to all kinds of things that are happening around you. Being hyper-focused on only one thing means you will miss out. As you begin your cancer journey, resolve to give up the "fight" and embrace what is about to come because I know, from experience and stories shared here, that this will lead to an experience you will cherish for the rest of your life.

## I WILL CALL THE SHERIFF

After a thirteen-hour surgery, one of the things they do is insert a tube up your nose and down into your stomach – a nasogastric tube (or NG tube). Its appearance is a typical rubber tube that is placed so they can feed you, should you be unable to eat. It hangs out the end of your nose and is sutured in place (with a stitch to the end of your nose) so that it doesn't fall down into the stomach. I have always been a self-advocate for my own care and believe that patients, too often, defer to physicians because of the perceived (and sometimes real) lack of understanding about what needs to be done and what should be done as treatment. It's also true that knowing what questions to ask can be challenging.

I had been in the hospital for about a week and, being treated in a teaching hospital; it was not uncommon to see different residents on different days. On this particular day, my resident doctor came to my room, and I felt a little uncomfortable around this guy. While I don't think he was unpleasant, he seemed quite distant and a little egocentric. At any rate, he asked me questions about how I felt, did the typical examination by looking over my incision site, and then proceeded to *tell* me that he was going to start feeding me through the NG tube because I was not eating enough food. I've never been a big fan of someone telling me what to do, so that was his first mistake. As we talked, he quickly figured out I was not happy. Certainly, I would not be opposed to treatment if it was going to help me. But after the discussion with him, I decided that I was not ready to be fed through the NG tube. In my mind, I had not been given enough time to try and take in more calories on my own. I don't remember exactly what he said, but I recall him trying to assert his authority over me, and so, in that moment, I looked at him and said, "If I have to call the sheriff, I will. You are not going to feed me through the NG tube."

The sheriff? Really? I'm not sure where that came from, but I just remember feeling vulnerable. He wasn't listening to me, and I needed him to stop and hear me. He did. What we ultimately agreed to was a one-day reprieve. I agreed to work hard to start eating more, and he agreed to hold off for one more day.

Over the next twenty-four hours, I worked hard to eat

as much as I could. The hardest part about recovering from my surgeries was always the process of starting to eat. The pain I felt when ingesting food was excruciating, and, ultimately, that led to real fear when sitting down to the table. Even though I was starting to eat more, I reluctantly agreed to allow the NG tube feeding to begin the next day. At my core, I knew it was the wrong decision, but I had made the deal and felt that I needed to try.

They pumped a thick, liquid food into the NG tube, and I remember, quickly, feeling the pain in my abdomen. It was reasonable to think that if food caused discomfort in my stomach, this wouldn't be any different. Looking back, I think that was the one question I forgot to ask – and certainly the one thing the physician neglected to consider, as well. When you are feeding yourself and have pain, you can stop eating, taking a break to allow food to settle. Having food pushed into your stomach by a pump, attached to a tube, takes away any control. My pain increased as the liquid kept being forced into my stomach. I was so uncomfortable and experiencing a vulnerability unlike anything I'd ever had.

Before I went into the hospital, I always said I could take almost any kind of pain that might be the result of a treatment. The only thing that I did *not* want to happen was for me to vomit. I hate to vomit. I know that most people, of course, don't enjoy it, but for some reason, that has long been the one thing I despise most. You have to understand that my incision was virtually as long as it could be up and down my abdomen, having opened me up as far as they could. Any use of abdominal muscles after surgery is incredibly painful. The body knows what it wants – and it did not want food in my stomach. Lying in my bed, I proceeded to vomit all over myself and was gagging on an NG tube that was coming out my throat but still sutured to my nose. The tube that was once down in my stomach had now come out when I vomited, so it went from my nose (where it was sutured) out through my mouth. It's incredibly difficult to try to breathe when you are choking on something.

It may seem crazy, but in that moment when I was gagging on a tube stuck in my throat, I can honestly tell you that I experienced one of the most joyful moments of my life. You see, I made a commitment before I started chemo the first time, to look for joy in the most excruciating moments. Because of the intention I had worked on for so long, I was able to take a step back from that painful experience, in that moment, and see what was happening around me. On my right was my sister, Tami. And as I gasped to catch my breath, I heard her yell out to a nurse, "We need a suture kit." She was calm and collected and knew exactly what to do because she is a trauma nurse. But that assurance of action was not what changed my life. It was the connection we made in that scary moment. I knew I wasn't going to die; I was just really uncomfortable, but as we waited for the arrival of scissors to cut the sutures securing that tube to my nose, I looked into my sister's eyes and saw and felt a love that I won't ever forget. I have always been close to my sister. In that moment, however, we cemented a relationship and bond that will be with me forever.

I've alluded to the fact that I was a real self-advocate during my treatments. With a few exceptions, during times when I was not capable, I always managed to maintain control of the treatment being administered to me. I wanted to understand what was happening, why it was happening, and what benefits I expected to see. Usually, I asked what might happen if I didn't do a certain procedure as well. In this case, I managed to maintain control but still had unintended consequences. Nevertheless, I experienced joy, in a moment of fear – because I chose to look. If you have the courage to stop fighting and embrace what follows in this book, I believe you can also find joy in moments where you never imagined it could exist.

3

# SHARE YOUR STORY AND YOUR JOURNEY

When first diagnosed with cancer, the urge to keep it secret and not be a burden is one that many people wrestle to overcome. In fact, I would venture to guess that most people never overcome this obstacle as the fear of being a burden to anyone is so prevalent. I think one of the mistakes made by many cancer patients is not letting others help. But the truth is, not allowing others to help is depriving them of an opportunity to be connected to you and feel that they are part of your life.

Additionally, you are missing out on opportunities to connect with people when you make the decision to self-isolate during your treatment. Frankly speaking, carrying the burden alone is not what you would want friends to do so it begs the question: why are you doing it? In my mind, not allowing others to help is a selfish thing for cancer patients to do. I remember a specific scenario during my first cancer diagnosis that helped me understand early on that cancer, in fact, affected more than just me. While I might be the one going through the treatment, it became crystal clear that others were also in pain.

## IT'S NOT JUST ABOUT ME

During my first diagnosis and treatment, chemotherapy hit my body like a ton of bricks. After only a month of treatment, my oncologist told me I had to stop eating. I went on TPN (total parenteral nutrition) and was fed through a needle for five months. Each evening, a gallon of nutrition would come out of the fridge, and it had to be prepared. Vitamins were added, and the tubes that connected the machine to the port in my chest had to be set up. I wanted to do this prep work myself in order to have the smallest sense of independence, but my mom, having also learned how to do it, was usually steps ahead of me and got it done before I had the chance. Being so dependent on others for so many things, I felt deprived of this opportunity to be self-sufficient. Even if it was something simple like preparing my own TPN, I wanted to do it. In the end, however, I realized that it made my mom happy when I allowed her to help. The simple act of preparing my nutrition gave her a purpose and made her feel needed. Given her normal love language of feeding people, I came to understand that this was her trying to be a part of my experience. I quickly realized that she would rather be the one going through chemotherapy rather than the one seeing the damage that chemotherapy was doing to her son.

Additionally, I had lived in my home in California for almost three years when my parents came to live with me. My backyard was still empty – no grass, no shrubs, no trees. In the five months that my parents lived with me, my backyard was transformed into a sanctuary with a gorgeous citrus tree, tons of shrubs, and an underground irrigation system on a timer that would ensure nothing would ever die. It also became clear that my dad needed to feel helpful.

They always took me to chemotherapy and church on Sundays. But in the end, I learned that people really do want to be a part of what is happening. I learned to sit back and allow others to help while looking at the situation from the other person's perspective. When someone I know is hurting, I don't see them as a burden but rather as an opportunity to step forward and help. And so, it was a lesson to me: I was not a burden. And I allowed others to help.

As you navigate your cancer journey, I encourage you to look at the situation from a friend's perspective. If your friend was feeling weak and needed a ride to chemotherapy, would you want to take them? Would you want to prepare a meal so your friend, feeling weak from chemotherapy, could rest and not have to cook? If the answers are yes, then open up and realize the possibility that you now have in your life. You have the opportunity to help people feel useful and feel like a part of something that they *want* to be a part of. Shutting people out and enduring things alone denies them the opportunity to feel useful and connected to you. In life, there are really only three things that matter (in my humble opinion): Love, Joy, and Connection. Many of the stories in this book are all about opportunities that arose because I had cancer. If I had been unwilling to share my journey, the love, the joy, and the connections I made would not have been possible.

Cancer is not just about you. Every decision you make will touch the lives of all those that love you. Vulnerability breeds a depth to life that you may not have seen or understood before this diagnosis. Allow yourself the opportunity that cancer has provided – open yourself up to others and let them help.

# 4

# FIND A WAY TO CREATE YOUR OWN EPIPHANY

Overcoming fear and pain does not happen magically. In fact, you will always find moments where the fear overcomes you, and the pain is more than you think you can bear. Not acknowledging this reality would be unfair and, in my opinion, doesn't serve you or the experience you are about to face. That said, there are ways to keep the fear and pain "in check." Many people believe in the power of meditation and prayer; others find that regular exercise and a good diet will help foster positive energy that will facilitate a more tolerable chemotherapy journey. While I agree these things can help, there is one thing that will help more than anything else: creating an intention to see something good in the most awful moments.

Countless books have been written on the power of intention when it comes to all kinds of topics: work, relationships, faith, life, happiness, and even life in general. As you navigate cancer and chemotherapy, it is my hope that you will summon up the courage and energy to find an intention for one thing and one thing only: seeing the joy in the worst parts of what is about to come.

At this moment, I want to challenge you to look inside yourself and find the space to recognize that joy does, in fact, exist in the same moments where fear and pain live. People often focus solely on the fear or pain, thereby ignoring, or simply not seeing, the joy that is also there in that same moment. Take a few minutes right now to recognize this fact. Having created this intention myself, I know that it can be life-altering. If you can find a way to move toward intention, I know the rewards will be more than you ever imagined. As you embark on your journey to begin chemotherapy, you know there will be scary moments. Remind yourself right now that you will commit to looking outside that space of fear and anxiety to see the joy that is right there, as well. This doesn't mean that chemotherapy will be joyful. It simply means you will *choose* to *look* for something joyful. I can't guarantee you will always find it, but the first step in seeing something good is creating a solid intentionality that will be with you throughout the cancer experience.

Nothing in my logical mind could have prepared me for the epiphany I was about to have on a beach in Spain. Anticipating chemotherapy is an agonizing trip that most cancer patients take with trepidation. Fear of the unknown and the anxiety that accompanies that fear is overwhelming, to say the least. I understand the need and the want to just "get it over with" so life can return to normal again. As you have likely heard before, life really is about moments, as most of us don't remember days. Moments are all you have. And yet, the prospect of undergoing chemotherapy makes people want to wish away time because treatment has nothing to offer but pain. In the following stories, my hope is to show you that finding a way to become intentional about your upcoming cancer journey can have major and consequential effects on what you are going to experience. I know, from experience, that this epiphany changed not only the course of my treatment – but my life. Stop now and create your intention to seek out joy as you forge ahead. Make a decision now to not simply wish away the time you will spend in treatment. Make a decision now to not simply live for a future time when all this is over. Make a decision now to look outside the upcoming moments of pain and see the good that is right there in that same moment.

## THE SPAIN TRIP

With the approval of my surgeon and oncologist, Bernie and I headed off to Spain in October 2004 to attend the wedding of a friend. I felt better, and my surgical incision had healed nicely though I had made the mistake of walking hunched over for several weeks after surgery; it was an instinctive mistake made to protect my abdominal area. However, it resulted in the scars healing "short," as it were. The scar tissue now needed to be stretched out, and that was a bit uncomfortable. Nevertheless, I was off to Spain with Bernie and determined to have a great vacation, knowing that upon my return life would be horrible as chemotherapy was going to begin.

My biggest problem, however, was related to the fact that I had recently lost part of my lower small intestine and part of my upper colon. And, unbeknownst to me, there is this little valve between the two called an ileocecal valve. Apparently, this valve closes off the colon from the small intestine so your body can absorb the nutrients in the small intestine. Once all the nutrients are absorbed, this little valve opens up and allows the waste material into the colon, where it is then excreted. Having lost this little control valve, my food went quickly through my small intestine and into my colon. This presented a problem in that I often needed to use the bathroom and was not provided much notice. I had a newfound empathy for anyone ever having to deal with ulcerative colitis or Crohn's Disease. But again, I was bound and determined to make this trip a good one.

I was in Barcelona and wanted to walk the city and see as much as we could. Unfortunately, walking made my problem worse, so we opted mostly for bus tours. We did, however, walk around Sagrada Familia, the largest church in the world currently under construction. It has been under construction since 1882 and was incredibly amazing to view in person. Imagining the changes in building techniques from when the cathedral started construction to the modern day was something I pondered in the large open spaces. The detail and magnificence of this structure were absolutely breathtaking. On the wedding day, I have amazing memories of the day and the reception following the ceremony. In fact, on the night of the wedding, it seemed as if my body was as it used to be. It was a moment when I wondered about the power of circumstances. It was as if my body reacted to the positive energy of the wedding space, and the celebratory atmosphere made me forget that I was still recovering from surgery.

Unfortunately, the Spain trip was, for the most part, one of the most difficult vacations I have ever taken. I'm certain that I was not good company as I was miserable much of the time. Additionally, I had such difficulty sleeping that my anger and discomfort were obvious. I resented Bernie during much of that trip because he was able to sleep just fine, and I couldn't sleep. I felt selfish and remember wondering how he could just go to sleep when I was unable to rest. My inability to communicate is obvious to me today, but unfortunately, it wasn't then, and Bernie took the brunt of my misplaced anger. Looking back, I was devolving into self-pity and didn't consider how my diagnosis and illness might have been affecting those around me. At this point, I hadn't quite embodied the notion that it wasn't all about me, and I certainly did not have the ability to see good things, for the most part.

MY EPIPHANY

While we were in Spain, Bernie's mom, Irene, and her husband, John, flew over to visit from England, where they lived. They visited for only a few days, but I know it was time Bernie cherished. With Bernie living in the United States, he didn't get to see his mom as frequently as he would like. I was glad she was able to meet with us since we were close.

Over the several days we spent together, Bernie and his mom were able to connect during much of the trip. We had lots of dinners together and spent quality time in conversation. On the day before Irene and John returned to England, it was unseasonably warm in Spain. I sat on the beach overlooking the Mediterranean Sea, and I saw Irene and John sitting at an outdoor cafe just up the beach while Bernie swam in the sea. The sun was bright blue with clouds in the sky, and the wind was softly blowing. Bernie was out in the ocean talking to strangers and reconnecting with friends he had not seen for a while. I've long believed that people don't remember days; they remember moments. This was a moment.

I opened my journal and wrote. As I turned inward to my thoughts, my initial writing was simply memorializing the trip to Spain and chronicling the agonizing moments I had endured during the trip as a result of my recent surgery. Journaling is often just a regurgitation of what's been done – and that's what I was doing. But as I continued writing, my words looked to the future. When I returned home, I would have outpatient surgery to have a catheter implanted in my chest. The following day, I would start a six-month chemotherapy treatment where I would be infused for almost three days straight, every other week. I wrote about how sick I might become and presupposed the worst possible scenario. I added language that supported my self-pity – specifically, noting the fact that I wouldn't be able to ski this coming winter. And then, still in pity, I wrote something that changed everything.

"I just want this to be over so I can move on with my life. I just want it to be May 2005 and then all this will be behind me."

I stopped. Sitting on the beach with sand between my toes and the sun shining brightly, I read that again. What was I doing? Was I really wishing away six months of my life? Did I really want the next six months to just disappear? I was in my mid-thirties and starting to understand the cliche that life goes by really fast. Suddenly, I realized that I didn't want to just wish away six months of my life. I couldn't do it. But what other choice did I have?

As I continued to capture the thoughts that raced through my mind, I recalled the words of my friend J.L.

"Nobody said life was fair, and nobody said it was easy."

And then I had the epiphany that changed the course of my chemotherapy and, ultimately, the course of my life. I wrote, "I will find joy in chemotherapy. In the midst of all that is purportedly bad, I will look, and I will see joy. I believe there is joy in the midst of this if I look."

I had a resolve that seemed to come from nowhere. Looking back, I know now there were events that led me to that moment – specifically JL's phone call and also Dr. Tracy's comment about skiing in South America. In that moment, I was no longer afraid, and I was no longer angry. I was going to live my life for the next six months, and my only mission was to find and see joy. And my strongest intention was to see joy in those moments when everything seemed the worst.

MY FIRST "JOY" MOMENT

It was the day after my epiphany on the beach, and it was the day that Bernie's mom would go back to England while Bernie and I would return to America. Little did I know that my first "joy" moment was about to occur at the airport when saying goodbye to Irene and John.

Bernie's mom adored her son. In July 2004, Bernie and I visited her in England and when she and John, her husband, picked us up at the airport, she just couldn't allow Bernard (she did not like that we called him Bernie) to sit in the back seat of the car. Consequently, I sat in the back seat with her while she chatted up Bernie (in the front seat) and ignored me. She seemed to do everything for him, short of cutting his meat before he ate. Okay, well, maybe I'm exaggerating a bit, but I have to say being around her was not easy for me. She doted on him in ways that were, frankly, uncomfortable. I'll admit that my own insecurities about gaining her approval may have been part of the issue, but, in my mind, it was clear that Irene just didn't like me. It seemed to me I made her uncomfortable, and I was also distracting her from her son, and she wanted his full and undivided attention.

In all honesty, I really loved Irene. There was an "air" about her, I recall. She exuded this energy and confidence that intrigued me. Of course, her lovely and sophisticated

British accent may have had something to do with it as well. But lest you think I'm awful, it should be noted that I really did have a great respect for Irene. I knew she missed her son and didn't get to see him nearly as often as she liked. But I still had this underlying feeling that she didn't want me around.

We all gathered in the entrance of the airport in Spain when we had to part and say goodbye. As we stood there, casually engaging in small talk as we allowed the minutes to tick away, I could tell she did not want to say goodbye. I have had this same experience with my own mother, many times, as it is always hard to leave knowing you won't see each other for several months again. Finally, she and Bernie hugged and kissed as they shared an emotional goodbye. I stood by, awaiting what I perceived to be my obligatory hug and goodbye from Irene. It always made me a bit nervous because it was uncomfortable, and remember, I really didn't think she liked me. What happened next totally surprised me. Irene stepped away from Bernie and turned toward me. As I reached out to give her a polite goodbye hug, she stopped me. She placed her hands on my shoulders, looked me square in the eyes, and said: "Kipp, I think about you every day, and I pray for you every day." That look. Those words. Joy.

There it was. Only yesterday, on the beach, did I decide to make an intention to look for joy in chemotherapy. Here it was; it had come early. In a moment where I faced a woman I thought despised me, my world changed. I had judged Irene unfairly, failing to see her for who she really was – a mother who dearly loved her son and was disconnected from him by an ocean. And she loved me. The words she spoke were insignificant compared to the feelings expressed by her connection with me in that moment. I felt an absolute and unconditional love from someone I thought did not care about me. I felt ashamed of myself for judging her so harshly, and more than that, I felt joy. As Irene walked off, I knew that I could find joy not just in chemotherapy but in all sorts of improbable places. I was now on a mission.

Over the next three years, I would have two cancer recurrences, which involved two additional thirteen-hour surgeries and more chemotherapy. This book contains the stories of moments where I saw joy – felt joy – because I chose to look. And it started almost after making the connection between intention and joy.

As you embark on your journey, I challenge you to recognize that there is joy in all kinds of unexpected and improbable places – but you have to be intentional and look for it. If you make a decision in *this* moment that you will look for something beyond the pain and uncomfortable parts of what is about to come, I guarantee you will create moments in your life that will outlast any fear or pain. People don't remember days; they remember moments.

Finally, I want to make sure you understand that fear is a part of this process. Making a commitment to finding joy amidst the pain doesn't mean the pain stops, and it doesn't mean the fear goes away. Accepting and recognizing the reality and truth of your experience and feelings is an important part of finding and creating your own epiphany. Even after going through chemotherapy and surgery twice, I still had fear, but I never let it distract me from also seeing and finding joy.

### I'M SCARED. ARE YOU?

In October 2007, after being diagnosed with cancer for the third time, I met Jane Stone in an online support group. I had met others in these forums, but Jane and I just connected for some reason. We chatted on the phone and ultimately, she came to North Dakota for a consultation with my surgical oncologist. When she flew in, we finally met in November, and I had dinner with her and her ex-partner, Linda, a woman with whom she shared custody of two daughters. I loved both of them and was amazed at how they were still supportive of each other. Though they no longer lived together, they had a connection that was incredible. Sharing children, their lives seemed to be built around ensuring these two girls were, in no way, pawns in some ongoing struggle. They loved each other but were no longer in love.

After having dinner, I went home and would often speak to and email Jane as she continued to weigh her options and determine what the best course of treatment was for her situation. I'm a positive and optimistic person by nature; Jane had a similar approach. Our emails often outlined the course of treatment recommended, what kind of recovery might be expected, and the side effects that may be experienced. Toward the end of November 2007, I received a lengthy email from Jane, as she had recently read some things on my blog and commented on those entries. In addition, she seemed to have entered the anger stage (which I believe is fairly typical for recent cancer patients) and was venting about the way she was being treated and how she had to hold her tongue around friends and family even though she knew their actions were coming from a place of love. She was venting her anger, and I got to be the sounding board. The email was, in most ways, unremarkable – and frankly, it rambled on a bit. But the last words of her email stuck with me: "I'm scared, are you? Love you, Jane."

Everything in that email – except those last words –

became irrelevant. Amidst her angry yet positive, optimistic attitude was a person genuinely scared of the unknown. She was a mother to two teenage daughters and was determined not to show them her fear. But those words, almost lost in the massive and lengthy email – I'm scared, are you – struck a chord with me. In a moment, I felt more connected to Jane than ever. Looking back, I feel more blessed since Jane, and I had only met a little more than a month prior to this email. Cancer connected us and if not for her diagnosis and mine, I would not know this amazingly beautiful woman.

Ultimately, Jane decided to have surgery on the East Coast, closer to her home in New Jersey. I would have my third surgery on December 5 and Jane would have her first surgery on December 27. Recovery from a thirteen-hour surgery and chemotherapy is not easy but this time, Jane and I did it together. Having support from someone who understood what I was going through was a new experience for me. As the months passed, we both became stronger, and life returned to its normal – absent cancer – state.

In October 2008, Jane came back to North Dakota for another visit. This time, she stayed with me, and there was no talk of doctor visits and cancer. I had a party at my home in honor of her visit. I asked Jane if having alcohol at the party would be a problem since she had been in recovery for many years. She assured me it would not be an issue. The party ended up getting a little out of control as some younger acquaintances showed up, blatantly drunk. Jane was always candid and honest about how she felt, and as we began cleaning up after all the guests left, she asked if I could take her to an AA meeting in the morning. Her honesty about how that party made her feel was such a lesson for me. I was embarrassed and ashamed of myself for allowing the party to escalate as it did. Additionally, that was the first time I ever got a sense of what it must be like to be in recovery. Truth be told, I had never put much thought into how it must feel living in a world that sometimes seems to revolve around social drinking.

Jane had never been to Canada, and so, after some discussion, we decided to road trip it to Winnipeg, just for one night. Being in the car for the three-and-a-half-hour drive was so much fun – we really got to connect. Truth be told, the trip was horrible in many ways. We laughed about our dodgy accommodations, generously given to me by a friend who owns a condo in Winnipeg. And basically, we just got up the next morning – after arriving late the previous evening – and headed back to Fargo. Really, it was about saying Jane had been to Canada. On the return trip, she bought this little stuffed animal at the restaurant where we ate breakfast. She said the dog reminded her of my dog, Gartner, and she wanted it as a keepsake.

On the trip home, she told me about the trip she and Linda took to China many years ago. They were there to adopt a daughter. In those days (and perhaps still today, I'm not sure), two women could not adopt a daughter together, so as they were getting all the paperwork together, the person with the adoption agency asked if they each wanted to adopt. Without much thought, they decided to adopt two daughters. Hearing that story, I knew how lucky those girls were. She also told me about China and how she loved the beautifully crafted kimonos. She told me about the one she bought as a gift to give away upon returning home but still held onto it because it held such joyous memories. We talked about how a material object can sometimes be more than just a material object. We connected.

On some level, I think Jane knew she was not doing

well. Looking back, I can see that she was trying to fit as much into her life as possible, and, at that time, she knew she didn't have much time left. Jane died on June 21, 2009. Shortly before her death, I received a package in the mail and inside the package was the most beautiful kimono and a little, tiny stuffed animal that looked just like Gartner. I don't have a lot of possessions with which I can't part, but these two are among my most treasured. Jane changed my life, and, to this day, she is part of who I am. And I'm a better person, having known her.

Acknowledging your fear and sharing it with someone you love can bring joy to your life and the life of another in ways you don't yet understand. Making the commitment to finding intention and exploring the possibility of being vulnerable will be the key to dealing with fear and pain. My hope is that by reading my stories of connection, you will find a way to create that epiphany that, I believe, you must have as you venture into the unknown.

5

# BEGINNING THE CHEMOTHERAPY JOURNEY

Having now found a way to an epiphany, I believe you are ready to begin chemotherapy with an understanding of how this journey can be more than just a painful experience. You are now equipped with intention and a new mindset that will positively shape what is about to come. Understanding there will be pain, fear, and perhaps some anxiety, you also know there will be joy along the way because of your intention to look for it from the beginning. When entering a new experience where consequences (most notably side effects) are unknown, it is easy to give in to negative emotions. Being intentional about the reality that joy exists in these difficult moments will be the catalyst that ensures you move through chemotherapy in a way that has lasting benefits in your life.

As I began my own chemotherapy experience, I was hyper-focused on finding joy in those really difficult moments, and, as you can see from the stories below, I found it time and time again. If you set intention as the focal point of your journey, I know you can have the same experience.

## SOME PEOPLE JUST "DO"

Susan Swiontek was probably my favorite teacher in high school. I met her in the seventh grade – it was her first year of teaching – and she was just out of college. She was an art teacher, so we all, of course, thought it was going to be a "slough" class; suffice it to say, we were all wrong. Mrs. Swiontek was a short lady and small in stature. I'm imagining that she probably would agree she overcompensated on that first day because she wanted to set the tone up front that she was not going to be a pushover. She would maintain discipline and have control of her class at all times.

Allowing others to help during chemotherapy is often a difficult thing for many patients to accept. Thoughts of being a burden and weak are often the excuses patients use to push away those who want to be there and support you. When you get diagnosed with cancer, it really is amazing the number of people who show up in your life from the past. People care. More than that, people really want to be a part of whatever it is that your diagnosis may bring. While few will see and understand the life-changing nature of a cancer diagnosis, that doesn't mean there aren't many who want to feel like they are a part of it. When cancer patients deny others an opportunity to help, they are taking away an opportunity for that person to feel helpful and needed. I'm certain you love the feeling you get when helping someone in need. Given this, denying people the opportunity to help you is, in my mind, much like snatching something away from that person. Often, people don't know what to do.

Add to that the fact that many of your loved ones are often hundreds or thousands of miles away, and you have a situation where people can easily feel disconnected. What surprised me was the people that didn't ask what they could do but simply did something and surprised me.

Seventh grade was a big year because as students, we were no longer saddled to a classroom with one teacher. This was the year when we moved from classroom to classroom. You started your school day in the locker room area chatting with friends, and then every class was held in a different room. This was a big deal. We entered art class in our daily rotation with the idea that we would be drawing, painting, and maybe doing some papier-mâché. When Mrs. Swiontek passed out a syllabus for her class, we all knew that art was not going to be easy.

At the time, I probably didn't realize it, but she was fresh out of college. She was young. She wanted to make sure we knew she was the boss. She was a small lady but tough; she didn't smile a lot and was, frankly, almost unfriendly. It was clear there would be no disciplinary problems in her class. She told us about the tests we would be given throughout the semester. Tests? In art class? This lady was crazy. In fact, she was an amazing teacher. She taught us about the primary and secondary colors by having us tap into our creativity. We learned about drawing three-dimensional objects by doing it. Over the course of that semester, she lightened up. But it was always clear she would have respect.

Mrs. Swiontek was also the yearbook advisor. With a real interest in photography, I joined the yearbook staff and forged a friendship with her over the course of my high school years. While in high school, I suppose we weren't really friends as she was always my teacher. Not until I was diagnosed with cancer did I realize that we really were friends.

I received a package in the mail one day, and when I opened it, I found the softest, most amazing Afghan, with a note from Susan. (I get to call her Susan now.) When I pulled the blanket from the box, it was as if I could feel the love in the softness of the yarn. She heard, through mutual friends, that I was diagnosed with cancer and knitted it just for me. Joy was showing up even before I started chemotherapy. I believe that absent my intention to look for and seek out joy; this may have simply been construed by me as a friend doing something nice. Instead, I recognized it and appreciated it for what it really was: Susan wanted to be part of my upcoming journey. And the only thing she knew to do was knit me an Afghan. In fact, that Afghan covered me for months as I often was cold during treatment. Recognizing the importance of allowing others to help is a bedrock of finding something good in the experience you are about to endure.

I'm certain she knew that her thoughtfulness would be appreciated. What I don't think she knows is how that act of unsolicited kindness stuck with me, even as the years have passed. Chemotherapy was not easy. But when wrapped in an Afghan, knitted by someone that helped shape my character, I felt safe. I felt loved. I felt joy – right from the beginning.

## GARTNER: DON'T TELL ME DOGS CAN'T COMMUNICATE

Gartner was my first dog, as an adult. He was, of course, named after Vi Gartner, my friend and my parents' bookkeeper. We had a dog, Mitzi, when I was a child and adolescent. But, at that age, I think we all tend to be self-involved and so the experience of having a dog in adulthood is much different. I loved Gartner more than I can possibly convey.

He was smart and always listened. I never wanted a dog that could do fancy tricks. I just wanted him to listen. Gartner listened. That is, until he was older. It was kind of funny. As he got older, you could almost see the wheels spinning in his head. If I said "sit," he would just look at me, as if to say, "yeah whatever, been there done that, I'm out of here." Then, he would turn and walk away. I think he figured he had been obedient for enough years, and he just wasn't having it anymore.

Gartner was a Bichon Frise, a French "lap dog." Purportedly, these dogs are snuggly and like to be held a lot, but this was certainly not true of Gartner. When he was younger, he used to run to the door to greet me when I would arrive home. Later in life, I think that ended mostly because he just couldn't hear, but I also believe he just couldn't be bothered. Honestly, he wasn't all that excitable, and I can recall many times when I would walk into the living room, and he would be lying on the couch just ignoring me. I would greet him and then sit on the opposite end of the couch. He would look at me, almost irritated, get up and go lay somewhere else. He would usually stay in the room and lay on the floor but just was not a dog that wanted to be too close to me, most of the time.

He did sleep on my bed at night, but he rarely slept next to me as he had his spot at the foot of the bed. I suppose he was independent – like me, I guess. In that way, he and I really connected. I knew he loved me, and he knew he was loved. If I ever picked him up to cuddle, he would endure it, though I knew he was just waiting to be put down again. I had come to terms with him not being a super affectionate dog and that was okay.

Alta Bates Herrick Campus in Berkeley, the chemotherapy unit where I had my first treatment in November 2004, was really a thriving place full of love and energy, which, in the beginning, seemed odd as people were being treated for cancer. In many ways, it exuded positive energy in a way we just don't see in everyday life. The nurses were all incredible, and, knowing that it was going to be my home away from home for the next six months, I felt good about my decision to have treatment there. After completing my infusion at the clinic, I was connected to a portable pump that would continuously administer a different chemotherapy drug over the course of the next forty-eight hours. I left the clinic and wore this pump over my shoulder, returning later to have the needle and pump removed so that I could begin my recuperation period.

My parents and I got home and quickly after getting my pajamas on, I felt weaker. The drugs were beginning to take their toll, so I grabbed my Afghan – the one given to me by my seventh-grade art teacher, Susan – and cuddled up on the sofa. Mom was in the kitchen preparing dinner and Dad was probably working on something around my house that needed fixing. As I laid there, my mind wandered. Would I soon get sick? Would I be able to sleep tonight? How would these drugs affect me? It was my first chemo session and there were so many unknowns. As my mind raced, Gartner jumped up on the sofa. I laid on my side and he cuddled right up next to me, snuggling into my chest. Is this my dog, I thought? What is going on?

As I petted Gartner, I felt love. And joy. There it was again. This time, from a dog. I am convinced that he knew I was sick. As tough as it was for him to be cuddled, he allowed it in that moment. And that's a moment I will never forget. In fact, I remember yelling to my mom, "Oh my gosh … Mom … look … Gartner is lying with me." She grabbed her camera and snapped a picture. Now I have that photo of him cuddling with me tattooed on the back of my leg. It was a moment I will never forget. And I believe intention is the reason I was able to create that moment. As you begin your chemotherapy treatment, remembering to look for the good things will have lasting, lifetime consequences. I was tired and weak in this moment, but because of my intention, I shared a moment with my dog that was out of character and rare.

## LAVINIA

Having now been through a couple rounds of chemotherapy, I determined that I was a wanderer. I was always anxious for the nurses to start my chemotherapy so I could get up and walk the halls of the Herrick Campus. Sitting in a chair while cell-destroying chemicals entered my body was not my idea of a good time. I needed to walk with my drugs in tow on the chemo pole and connect with people. That's what life is about for me. Even in a place that's supposed to be sad and depressing, I was constantly on the lookout for joy.

This is how I met Lavinia. My beachside epiphany was foremost in my mind, so I was determined to find joy. Perhaps that is why I had to wander. Sitting in the chair, joy wasn't coming to me, so I decided to get up and find it. The chemo ward was set up with private rooms on the outside and groups of chairs on the inside. The chairs were for those of us who were able to tolerate chemo more easily. The private rooms had beds, and those patients often experienced the worst side effects and so were granted additional space, comfort, and privacy.

Walking by her room that day, I remember seeing Lavinia in her bed – alone. She was awake and our eyes met. I'm generally not the person who approaches others to chat, but, on this day, her eyes seemed to say, "come on in." So, I did. She was smart – and better yet; she was intelligent and well-spoken. She was artistic and well-read with varied interests. Being near her gave me a sense of connection to the world – both past and present. We talked endlessly, and in a small amount of time – almost – I knew who she was, and I knew I loved the kind of person she was in the world. She had a way of putting me at ease, and, looking back now, it's easy for me to understand why we connected. As we both endured the toxic drugs that were entering our bodies, we found something good. Maybe in some way, we simply distracted each other from the reality of our situations. It really was more than that, though. I know it was joy and new friendship that we found in that moment on that day. I wandered. I looked. And there it was – Joy.

Over the weeks and months that followed, Lavinia and I developed a real friendship. Interestingly enough, the relationship reminded me of the one I had with Vi Gartner years earlier. Lavinia and I didn't see each other outside of Herrick Campus. However, while there, we managed to forge a relationship that I know we both cherished. I believe Lavinia was seventy-eight years old, and so, it proved to be difficult for her to tolerate the chemotherapy treatments. She often spoke of her home and how she just wanted to be there. She lived with her twin sister – I think her name was Polly, but I'm not sure – and they were extremely close. As Polly cared for Lavinia, I would watch and think of my own brother and sister. Would I care for Tami at age seventy-eight? Would I care for Todd in this way? Would they care for me? It was so interesting to watch. There it was again. Joy. I was paying attention, and it showed up.

Lavinia and I went through nearly six months of chemotherapy together. During that time, we had many conversations and just as many moments where we simply sat together quietly. She was often tired, and it became difficult for her to muster the energy to engage in conversation. I remember a particular moment toward the end when I saw her in the waiting room. She was sitting in a wheelchair and her sister, Polly, was in a chair next to her. This moment – though I didn't know it at the time – would become a defining moment in my life.

I saw her come in and, after a few moments, I walked over to say hello. She was weak; in fact, I had never seen her with so little energy. I knelt down on the floor so she didn't have to look up at me. She was in her wheelchair, almost hunched over as if even sitting was a chore. We exchanged hello's and, sensing her weakness, I just decided to talk so she didn't have to engage with me. I told her a story about something my sister and I had recently discussed. Frankly speaking, I don't remember the story I told; but I do remember how I told it. Referring to my sister, I said something like "… her and I went to this party …" As I rambled on with my story, her weak and frail arm lifted up and started gently tapping me on the shoulder. When I think of this moment, it's as if I can still feel that gentle, loving tap on my shoulder. It continued. She just kept tapping until I stopped talking. When I eventually stopped to listen, she looked in my eyes and quietly echoed the words "It's she and I … Kipp, it's she and I …" In that moment, with barely enough energy to maintain an upright posture in a wheelchair, Lavinia corrected my grammar.

This is why I loved Lavinia, and this exemplifies who she was. She didn't want me to wander through the world using improper grammar, so she corrected me even when she barely had the energy to sit up. To this day, whenever I am faced with a situation where I need to use these pronouns, Lavinia Holmquist is alive and well. She lives in me and through me. I carry her with me forever and ever. She touched my life and changed me in a moment. And she never knew it. Paying attention during treatment will be one of the hardest things you do as side effects distract you. Giving in to the thing that has the most control – pain – is the easy approach. Focusing on intention in all situations can be the difference between finding joy and finding pain.

## YOU NEED TO MAKE A LIST

There was one time – only one – when they were not able to be with me. My sister, Tami, got engaged and was married during a small ceremony in December 2004. The wedding reception, however, was going to be in January 2005. I insisted my parents stay in North Dakota following Christmas, so they could be there for Tami. Unfortunately, I had to return to California, where I would continue my treatment.

I got home and was there alone, with my dog. I felt a little like life was normal again. My parents living with me during chemotherapy was loving and supportive, but this brief glimpse into what my life used to be was eye-opening and drastically needed. My chemotherapy was timed so that I was feeling well enough to fly home to North Dakota over the Christmas holiday. When I returned, I had a few days before I had to check myself into the hospital for chemotherapy. The treatment affected me to the point where my oncologist wanted me in the hospital for the three-day infusion of chemotherapy. While in the hospital,

I seemed to tolerate the drugs better, with hydration being part of the routine.

Before I went into the hospital, Bernie and I planned a long weekend. He was going to fly in from Connecticut for the weekend and leave the day before I went into the hospital. At the end of a treatment cycle, I always had the most energy, so we tried to plan his visits around my schedule. Bernie lived in the east, and I lived in the west. We met in January 2004 while I was on my annual Whistler, British Columbia ski trip. I can't forget the moment when I met him. We just clicked. It seemed a little silly to try and date someone from England who was living in Connecticut while I was living in California. But it worked. We made it work, and we had an amazing first year.

Our relationship, however, wasn't without its faults. Now, with me being ill, the burden to travel was solely placed on his shoulders. Add that to all the other little issues, and our relationship was destined to fall apart. On the night before I was to go into the hospital and have three days of chemotherapy (without my parents' presence), Bernie and I decided to end our relationship. Honestly, it wasn't a big surprise, but I was hurt. I spent many years wondering how Bernie could leave me during a time when I was so vulnerable. I always imagined that I would have been the person who stayed, even though problems existed. I imagined I would wait until the other person was better to either resolve the issues or move on to something else. I'm grateful to say that I eventually came to terms with how our relationship ended, and I know why Bernie left when he did. To this day, he remains one of the people to whom I feel most connected.

In the morning, Bernie got a taxi to the airport, and I

headed off to Alta Bates Hospital where I would check in for three days of inpatient chemotherapy. My spirits were in need of a little lifting, to say the least. And, having been through chemotherapy in the hospital once already, I knew the road that was about to be traveled. My body would do better with nursing care around the clock, but it's never fun or easy being in the hospital. When I checked in, I sat on the edge of that hospital bed waiting for the charge nurse to come in and give me instructions. I looked around the room, gazed out the window at the gorgeous scenery, and thought about Bernie. How would I move through this without him? Did I make a mistake? What would tonight be like without a phone call to Bernie; we talked every night since we met nearly a year ago. I longed for his support and love, and in that moment, I missed him already.

In the midst of my pondering, in walked the charge nurse happier than she should be, in my opinion. With a giant smile on her face, she greeted me with what can only be described as perkiness, "And how are you doing today?" Without pause, I wimpishly said, "Well, I just got dumped by my boyfriend last night and I'm about to have three days of chemo. I've been better." Okay, yes, I was exaggerating. I hadn't really been dumped but I was looking for some sympathy. Luckily, this was a smart nurse (like most of them) and so she jabbed back at me in an instant, "You need to make a list."

What? A list? Truth be told, I knew exactly what she was saying. I had heard of this concept from other people. The idea is that you make a list with three columns: Must Haves, Would Be Nice to Haves, and Deal Breakers. In each column, you make a list of the characteristics of your ideal partner. Deal Breakers had to be exactly that – a Deal Breaker – no compromising. in that moment, this nurse managed to take me from a place of victimhood to empowerment. She said that this was the perfect time for me to make the list, as I would not be biased in any way. She reminded me that the list can't be made while dating someone. When she finished checking me in for my hospital stay, she left the room reminding me that she would be back the next day. She expected to see ten things on my list.

She did come back. And I still have the list. This moment was still in the beginning stages of my first bout with cancer, and this nurse refused to allow me to be a victim. Having the intention to look for and find joy is what, I believe, helped me see her as that source of joy and not someone who was being combative with me. It would have been easy to brand her as someone who was not empathetic with my situation. Most people would grant someone permission to mourn a lost relationship, especially when it had only happened hours ago. The creation of my intention in all parts of my chemotherapy journey allowed me to see her for what she was: love. I challenge you to continue to look for the good, even in the midst of the bad.

BOB

Whenever chemo was being pumped into my body, I felt the need to move around and wander the halls. I'm not sure why. But whether in the clinic or the hospital, I grabbed my chemo pole and wandered. In the early days of my first cancer treatment, I was admitted to the hospital for three days of inpatient chemotherapy. The drugs were not being tolerated by my body, so my oncologist wanted to figure out what was happening. In the hospital, the chemotherapy floor was set up in a sort of circle. You could literally walk all the way around the unit in a circle.

In the middle were the nurse's station and some offices. The patient rooms were all on the outside perimeter.

As I walked, I would stop, have a brief conversation with someone and then move on again. In three days, I managed to forge some temporary relationships. Bob was from somewhere near Lake Tahoe, and he was sick. I remember he had a sort of vestibule between the hallway and his hospital bed. It was a place for people to decontaminate themselves before going in to see him. He and I talked a lot over the course of my three days in the hospital.

Bob affected my life in ways he can't even imagine. You see, I have a real fear of conversations when in large groups. I'm not sure why. Part of it is the fact that I don't like to "compete" for conversation time. And it's a rare opportunity for me to meet someone with whom I can have conversations that just flow. I'm not good at small talk. I like big talk. I love pondering the universe and its purpose, discussing religion, discussing politics and socially accepted morality versus immorality. Life is too big for me to talk about the weather or celebrity culture. I understand some people revel in this, and I don't judge – it's just not who I am.

This is a guy who, in the midst of a severe cancer diagnosis, was an absolute joy. He once told me that he and his wife just had twins; she was home taking care of the babies, while he was in the hospital hundreds of miles from home. He was alone. So was I. Somehow, the universe put the two of us together.

He and I would talk for, what seemed to be, hours. In fact, we probably had brief conversation as both of us were undergoing chemotherapy. On my last day in the hospital, we were in my room chatting away. I knew that I would probably never see him again. With that in mind, I felt compelled to tell him how I had appreciated his friendship and companionship over the last few days. I believe I said something like, "Bob, I just want you to know that when I am talking with you, I feel like a person with knowledge. I feel like my voice is powerful. I feel like there's a purpose within me. You are amazing." And I will never forget his response. You see, I was giving him all the credit for how I was feeling empowered. He looked at me and said, "Kipp, I'm just a mirror reflecting back to you all that you are."

Bob was not the reason I felt powerful. But Bob is the one who reminded me that I can be as big or little as I choose. And later, I would learn that the people with whom we choose to surround ourselves may be as important as our message. We all need to see who we are, sometimes. Bob allowed me to see myself in a way I never had.

To this day, I don't know where Bob is. I don't know his last name. And I'm not sure I would recognize his face. But his spirit and his soul are connected to me. Forever.

### THE CALL FROM BRITISH COLUMBIA

As stipulated, I was not happy about missing my annual ski trip to British Columbia, with my friends. I started chemotherapy in November 2004 and by February 2005, I had the routine down cold. I would have chemo at the clinic in Berkeley during the day, return home and get forty-eight hours more of chemo from a pump that I wore over my shoulder, then I would endure at least a week of low energy, some nausea, and serious chills. I sat around in thermal pajamas and a cap while my dad wore shorts, and my mom wore her night gown. They sweated while I was freezing. At any rate, the routine usually allowed me a few days toward the end where I had enough energy to start moving about in the world again.

It was at the end of one of these chemo cycles in February 2005 when I ventured out with my parents to look at cars. They had driven back to California after Christmas so they could have a car to drive while living with me. My dad always hated their car; it was the first one my mom ever purchased without him, so I have a sense that may have had something to do with his dislike for the car. No matter, they had decided (or maybe it was Dad who decided) they were going to buy a new car while they were with me.

We spent the afternoon going from one dealership to the next, and I remember thinking about my ski buddies. It was the Whistler ski week, and they were all skiing and snowboarding at that moment. I was meandering around Oakland, looking at cars with my parents. My buddy, J.L., was calling. I knew he was in British Columbia, so I answered. I had been thinking about them all afternoon. What I heard on the other end of the phone when I answered was a group of people at Après Ski (the gathering in the bar after a long day of skiing), all greeting me and all thinking about me.

To this day, the thought of that moment brings tears to my eyes. These amazingly wonderful friends had just spent a day skiing in Canada. And at the end of the day, they raised a glass with positive energy flowing toward me. That call made me feel loved. And they don't know it. I could have felt sorry for myself in that moment, missing out on an annual trip I had taken for years with my friends. Truth be told, I had spent some time wallowing in pity because of what I was losing. That call, however, reminded me that sometimes life just looks different. Routines and patterns can be good but breaking up the monotony of life can sometimes be a good thing. I needed to be where I was in that moment to see that friendship can survive obstacles.

The beginning stage of chemotherapy and cancer treatment is the hardest. Navigating the complexities of treatment and presupposing whatever bad side effects might occur takes a lot of energy and focus away from what really matters. It's a natural thing that happens, and the only way to avoid this is by creating that intention to drive your focus elsewhere. I had shared stories of moments when things weren't so great. But in those moments, I was able to find something amazing and good because of my epiphany that created the intention to look for joy. As you navigate your journey, the beginning is the time when you will have to work the hardest to focus and shift your gaze to see all the good things that are happening. As I've noted many times, seeing joy doesn't always make the pain go away. That said, I can tell you this: having been cancer-free for many years, I don't remember or contemplate the painful moments. I remember and cherish the joyful ones. And if you don't look for joy, you don't get to cherish it in the years to come.

# EMBRACING THE CHEMOTHERAPY JOURNEY

Being in the midst of chemotherapy can wear on not only a person's physical well-being but mental state, as well. Beginning chemotherapy with an intention to seek out joy might be easier because you are not yet experiencing side effects from treatment. Your state of mind and commitment to intention will become increasingly important as you feel as if your body is giving up on you. Self-pity and defeatism will be easy coping mechanisms, but, rest assured, these are not strategies that will gain you any new perspective on your cancer journey or your life in general.

As your body begins to wane, be resolute. I believe if you reach into the inner parts of who you are and remind yourself of the intention you created when starting, you will continue to see and experience joy. Even when you find yourself annoyed or irritated, remember to allow the intention to distract you from that annoyance. In my experience, there is something else there, but you must take the time to look. Recalling stories from my own cancer journeys about times when I saw joy might serve as a reminder to you that it can happen. Continuing to hold space for intention is really the key.

## JILL, THE NURSE

I had lots of nurses treat me over the course of my cancer diagnoses, and I learned to value and trust the wisdom of nurses, oftentimes even more than physicians. They are in the trenches daily, and they see what works and what doesn't. I don't remember all the nurses who cared for me over the years, but I do remember Jill. She introduced herself, and I had a negative first impression of her. I had been getting chemo for several months, yet she had never treated me before this day. Most nurses had a loving character that was obvious and apparent, and perhaps I had become accustomed to that type of "bedside manner."

Jill had a British accent, long hair, and she was tough – a little rough around the edges, you might say. You could tell she was independent, the kind of person that didn't take grief from anyone, and I was irritated that day because of her unfriendly nature; she was a little short as if she was pressed for time. As usual, I got connected to my chemo and then started wandering the ward to begin chatting with other patients, but I found myself unusually frazzled because of my experience with her. Today, I look back on that experience and clearly see how victimhood was taking over in that moment for me. Jill didn't coddle me like some sick patient, but rather; she treated me directly and quickly. It really was more about me that day than it was about her.

Additionally, what strikes me today, and what struck me soon after that first introduction, is that I realized I was judgmental and unfair. Having Jill as my nurse many more times, I came to admire and love her. I learned that it was unfair for me to judge someone based on whatever preconceived ideas I had about how a nurse should treat a patient. Many of us have heard that first impressions are usually right, and I can attest to that often being the case. Jill, however, taught me that sometimes that is not the case.

I had several great nurses. Jill was one of them. I will always remember her because I initially judged her unfairly – and she reminded me that everyone deserves second chances. In fact, on my last day of chemo, Jill was the one who carried the flowers in that huddle of nurses. It was standing practice at Alta Bates Herrick Campus in Berkeley to present flowers to patients upon completion of their prescribed treatment. In my mind, I can see her smiling face now as the group of nurses walked toward me in the lobby that day. Jill is but one more example of a person touching my life – and she doesn't know it. As you encounter people during your cancer treatment, I would caution you to jump to conclusions as I did. My intention to look for joy failed me that day and it was a stark reminder of why it's important.

## WE LOST THE BATTLE, BUT THE WAR ISN'T OVER

I grew up in a town of approximately 1,300 people in North Dakota, and by many standards, it was a sheltered life. Having now lived all across the United States and traveled to several different countries, I know people are products of their environments. Even after leaving my small town many years ago, it still feels like home in some ways. In the 1980s, however, being a gay boy in a small North Dakota town was neither easy for me nor acceptable to anyone – at least not anyone I knew.

My parents owned a farm implement business, and I

recall hearing my dad say that "faggots should be locked up and the key should be thrown away." My mom had me and my brother and sister watch a Sunday night movie about a boy who came out to his parents. More vivid are the words she uttered at the commercial time: "I just don't know what I would do if one of you kids ever did that to us." As a child, I always knew I was gay, and I also knew it was wrong. It was a strange place to be as an adolescent – not knowing how to reconcile those inside feelings with what the world was telling me.

More than anything else, however, I was lucky to have parents that always preached about unconditional love over anything else. I heard those words – unconditional love – far more than any hateful language about gay people. Even though it was scary, I ultimately came out to them in August 1990. It was a long road to understanding and acceptance, but I believe our family is closer and stronger today because of my willingness to be honest with them in a time when it wasn't so easily accepted.

As my parents moved forward in the 1990s, they wrestled with telling friends about their gay son. As time went by, it became easier, and in fact, my dad told a story about one night when he was at a small-town bar and some guy was talking about gay people in a denigrating manner. He told me how he said to this person, "You don't know what the hell you're talking about." My dad told me this story years ago, and yet, still today, it is a moment that still evokes such strong emotions for me. It was the moment when I knew my dad understood ignorance and intolerance. In his voice, as he told the story, I could hear and feel his frustration and shame – shame for all the previous years when he was not so enlightened. I could tell stories of letters to the editor, written by my parents in support of gay people fighting for acceptance in their church. I could tell stories of my dad sacrificing income for their business because he didn't want to be associated with people who stood to infringe upon his son's rights. More important, however, are the stories about them simply acknowledging, to their friends, the fact that they had a gay son.

I know I had met Robbie Robertson on a few occasions. But the truth is, I really didn't know him well. I knew he was a great friend to my dad, and I knew they had talked about the fact that I was gay, but really, I didn't know much else about him. It was November 2004, and I had only recently begun chemotherapy. For some reason, I had a difficult time with the treatment, even though I was advised that most patients were able to continue working during my particular chemotherapy treatment. I had severe digestive issues and as a result, I lost weight. It was also an election year and the time when many states were passing constitutional amendments to define marriage as between one man and one woman. In North Dakota, an amendment was on the ballot, as well.

I was born and raised in North Dakota. If you're like me, I believe you probably feel forever connected to the place where you grew up. North Dakota was my childhood home and will, in many ways, be "home" forever. In my mid-thirties at the time, I had spent more than half my life outside the borders of North Dakota, but it was still home, and I longed for that place to recognize that a constitutional amendment was wrong.

I remember election night vividly. The chemotherapy had taken its toll on my body, and the election results of one state after the other approving constitutional amendments were making me feel as if America didn't care about me. I suppose I was being a bit of a victim. I don't think people, who aren't gay, can fully understand the feeling of having an entire country say to you, "You don't deserve equal rights. You deserve less." That night tortured me, and I was incredibly sad when I heard the news that North Dakota passed the amendment to define marriage as one man and one woman.

Shortly after this news was announced, I remember the phone ringing and hearing my dad chit-chatting for a bit. He then handed me the phone, and it was Robbie Robertson. He called to talk to me. When my dad handed me the phone, I was confused and perplexed. I didn't know Robbie that well, and yet he wanted to talk to me? He said, "Kipp, it looks like we lost the battle. But the war's not over. I'm sorry." In the blink of an eye, my victim mentality shifted, and I knew the world was changing. This man, who I was certain only years ago would have voted in favor of that amendment, was calling to apologize for something that really was not within his control.

Many years passed by, but the truth is, he was right about "the war." On June 26, 2015, the United States Supreme Court ruled on marriage equality for all people. I was in my car when I heard the news, and I called my mom and cried. Then, I had one more call to make. Robbie answered the phone, and he knew exactly why I was calling. Years before this moment, in the midst of chemotherapy, I found joy in a sad moment. On that day in my car, I found joy again – this time in a happy moment. Intention, as always, was the key.

## QS/1: A COMPANY WITH HEART

When I was first diagnosed with cancer in 2004, I had been working with a software company based in South Carolina for more than nine years. I started with them as a customer, having purchased the software for a drug store in which I was working. I joined the company in 1996 as a software trainer, and after only a couple of years, I moved into a sales position and then, three years later, took a role in management. I was responsible for eleven states on the west coast, as well as customers in Guam and Saipan. I oversaw three regional offices and, consequently, traveled quite a bit.

After beginning chemotherapy in November, it soon became clear that I was going to be unable to continue my role as Regional Manager during my treatment. I missed work, being too weak and too sick to leave home. It was frustrating to me that I appeared weak, but the reality of my situation was such that my body just couldn't do it all. After missing several days in the office, I received a phone call from corporate. I was advised that Bill Roberts, the human resources manager, would be coming to California to visit with me. I remember hanging up the phone and feeling a sense of fear. Was I going to be replaced? Was I going to be terminated? Flying in the manager of human resources from South Carolina seemed like a big deal.

I was not well enough to meet at the office, so I asked Bill to come to my home. He arrived with my boss, Ed Willett, the vice president of regional operations. I sat at my kitchen table just waiting for the bad news. Bill spoke and he talked about how it had become clear to them that I was going to be unable to continue in my role as regional manager. Crap. I can't believe this is happening, I thought.

As Bill continued speaking, I was dumbfounded. He said they wanted me to take whatever time I needed to get well. My health was the top priority and they wanted to visit with me so that I knew, firsthand, they were going to support me through this difficult treatment. They would continue to pay me. What? I was trying to keep my composure but found myself speechless, with tears. These two men, in that moment, brought a sense of relief to my world. I would no longer have to worry about losing my job. Or working. I could now focus all my energy on getting better.

I was looking for joy, all the time. And here it was – from a corporation.

## "DINNER" WITH A FRIEND

Unfortunately, my body did not tolerate the chemotherapy drugs during my first diagnosis and treatment. As noted previously, my oncologist had me do inpatient chemotherapy at a hospital to better control the side effects. After that, she determined that it would be best if I simply stopped putting anything into my digestive system during the next five months of treatment. With that advice, I began getting nourishment through the port that had been surgically implanted in my upper chest. The nutrition I would receive is called Total Parenteral Nutrition (TPN). Essentially, it is a gallon of liquid that gets administered over the course of twelve hours. I began the process each evening, and it would then be completed in the morning. A person can get used to almost anything, I suppose, but hunger is a difficult one. With nutrition being pumped directly into my bloodstream, my stomach remained empty. With an empty stomach, your brain thinks you're hungry. For most, this would be a terrible thing to endure. And it was a terrible thing; however, it also served as a constant reminder of how lucky and how grateful I want to be in every given moment.

I imagined being hungry and not having access to food. There, feeling pangs of hunger, was joy. Imagine living with your mom, having to smell the meals she cooked daily, but not being able to eat. It was a challenge. Almost every Sunday, I remember rewarding myself with three large green olives with pimentos. Oh, how I savored those three olives. I always knew I would pay for it with a stomachache, but I didn't care. To this day, even the sight of a green olive takes me back to those moments.

Most of my friends knew that I was not able to eat. That said, I didn't receive many dinner invites for the duration of my chemotherapy. My friend, Scott Thompson, however, is from Australia, and he didn't know any of this. When I received a call from him asking me to dinner, I was thrilled. He was traveling through San Francisco on his vacation and thought of me. I told him about my cancer diagnosis and so asked if he could come to my place and we would walk down to Piedmont Avenue, where we could find all kinds of restaurants.

When he arrived at my home, I informed him that I couldn't eat and had my bag of food already connected and over my shoulder. In a way, I think he felt badly that I was not going to be able to eat. By this time, however, I had become accustomed to watching other people eat. Ultimately, we decided on Jamaican food as we wandered up and down Piedmont Avenue. What makes this story so memorable for me is the sense of normalcy it brought to my life during that long period of time when life was so abnormal. I don't recall going out to dinner with anyone else while having TPN as my nutrition. I rarely see Scott, as he is from Australia, so this meal was especially memorable. Even today, I can close my eyes and picture the table in the restaurant, the corner in which we sat, the amazing conversation and it makes me smile. Scott's simple gesture, going out to dinner with me, interrupted what had become a monotonous life. And though I could not enjoy the food, that evening was a reminder of what life is really about. For me, it has always been about the connections I have to other people. That night, I connected with Scott, and he brought joy to my world. Joy, over a simple dinner invite.

## DR. TRACY DOES HAVE A HEART

From November 2004 to May 2005, I was being treated by Dr. Martha Tracy in Berkeley, California. As I've written, my parents didn't dislike her, but they were also not huge fans. However, I think they came to respect her a great deal as I moved through treatment. She was not an emotional support mechanism and was, in some ways, detached. I imagine treating cancer patients to be a really tough job, since not everyone gets better, and so I always suspected that she wore "tough skin" to protect herself and maintain a clear head. In fact, that was one of the things I really loved about her – the ability to think critically during times when things were not going as planned.

My treatment plan called for twelve rounds of chemotherapy, with each round lasting approximately three days. I was twice hospitalized because the drugs affected my digestive system harshly. After only a month of chemotherapy, I was forced to stop eating for the duration of my treatment and I would get nourishment through a port in my chest. Once I managed to get on a consistent routine, the treatments became more tolerable. I knew I would be sick, and I knew I would have virtually no energy for a certain period of time, but I also knew that I would get better. This is the reality of chemotherapy and it's one that I believe can serve patients well if they embrace it and understand it. If you know and understand how your body reacts (after the first treatment cycle), you can prepare yourself. Knowing you will get better is a great comfort in those moments when you feel awful.

Following treatment number eleven, I remember the

feeling of being close to the finish line. I remember thinking that I had just one more treatment to go. Then, during my post-treatment recovery days, my body gave out on me as the neuropathy in my hands and feet was no longer diminished by the time I was set to start treatment number twelve. My feet and fingers were numb, and it was becoming more difficult to walk. I was still weak and knew my body could not tolerate any more chemotherapy. After all I'd been through, I had finally learned to listen to my body, so I knew I could not proceed with the final treatment. Now, I needed to tell Dr. Tracy.

She could be tough, and I was nervous to tell her. When I arrived for my final chemotherapy appointment, I asked to see Dr. Tracy, which was not the usual protocol. Normally, I would just get started. I can still remember the feeling I had sitting in that consultation room, waiting for her to enter. It was as if she was my coach, having been cheering me on for almost six months and here I was throwing in the towel. I didn't want to disappoint her.

As she entered the room, she sat down and asked what my concerns were. I blurted out, "I have decided that my body can no longer take the side effects from chemotherapy. I'm done. I do not want to have treatment today." She looked at me, asked about my neuropathy, looked at the recent lab results in my chart and then put the file down, looked at me square in the eye and said, "I agree." The relief I felt was absolute joy. She stood up and extended her arms toward me and we hugged. For the first time in over six months, she showed me a side of her that I had not seen. I would have always been grateful to her, even had I left there with a handshake. But that simple gesture from her was a gift that I cherish. My sense is she can't possibly know what that meant to me. It was joy, from my oncologist, as I crossed the finish line – even if I finished a little early.

## FAMILY, MUSIC, AND A MOMENT THAT CONNECTED US ALL

Being in a hospital is never fun. But surprisingly, there are a lot of interesting and amazing things that happen in those places. I am always surprised at how willingly people give of their time and energy. Surgery usually happens in the early morning hours. With that said, I checked into the hospital the night before surgery, and I remember hanging out with my family the night before one of my operations. I had a small private room, and it was full of people. We were chatting when, out of nowhere, this girl appeared at the entrance to my room. She had a guitar and wanted to know if we would be interested in some music. We couldn't say no.

As she played, all the talking stopped, and we were focused solely on her. She had power in that moment. She was confident and made every effort to make eye contact with me, the patient. She sang and looked into my eyes. That kind of attention and direct eye contact can sometimes make me nervous. But she didn't. In those few minutes, while she played and sang, I was once again reminded that this process that I was about to begin (yet again) was going to be filled with joy. I had been through surgery and chemotherapy before and knew that joy existed in those moments. And as I stared into her eyes, I felt comforted. Joy – from a stranger.

## JHAY MACGREGOR

Based on all the time I've spent in hospital beds and chemotherapy units over the years, I have come to various conclusions about the state of our healthcare system. Overall, I have been extremely fortunate. First off, I'm thorough and I ask lots of questions. Secondly, I've been lucky to have great health insurance each time. When I was first diagnosed, I was so lucky to work with a company that supported me and allowed me the time off to get better. Absent that, I'm not sure I could have handled it. When faced with a life-threatening illness, people should not have to worry about how they are going to pay for the treatment. Luckily, I did not have that stress.

One of the other things I learned is that we all need to listen to our bodies more often. Prior to my first diagnosis, I knew something was wrong. But having gone to see my primary care physician, she ruled out anything major. I trusted her. And, frankly speaking, she is an incredible physician, and I don't fault her at all. Had I been more assertive, she may have taken the situation further and diagnosed me a few months earlier. Of course, with my history, they now throw me in a CT scanner if I complain about a sore toe. I suppose that's a benefit to having my medical history.

The observation that has struck me the most, however, is that nurses really are the backbone of care when you are sick. Nurses, not physicians, were almost always the ones who treated me and made me feel better. As with any rule, however, there can be exceptions.

My surgical oncologist was Robert Sticca and he, too, made me feel better and always provided the information that I wanted as a proactive patient. I have great respect for him and recall his visits to my hospital room at the earliest hours of the morning. One of the things I liked about Dr. Sticca was that he almost always came to my room alone, early in the morning. He would come again later, with a slew of interns. Jhay MacGregor was one of the students working with Dr. Sticca. Jhay MacGregor was exceptional.

The first time Dr. MacGregor stopped by to see how I was doing, I was a little dumbstruck. Having spent a good amount of time in the hospital, I knew this was out of the ordinary. My cancer was rare, and the treatment, at the time, was even more uncommon. I considered that maybe he, as a student, had a medical interest in my case. After he continued showing up, I realized it was more than a simple interest in my medical case. Dr. MacGregor was always on rounds with the group. He would then stop back in, later, by himself. While not daily and not often, it was enough for me to realize that this was a guy who was on his way, without a doubt, to becoming an outstanding physician. Not surprisingly, today he is chief of surgery at a veteran's hospital.

I can't even really explain to you what it was about him. He asked me to call him Jhay. A young doctor, in a learning hospital, stopping by to say hi. A young doctor breaking down that wall of superiority by simply asking me to call him Jhay. That wall can sometimes make patients feel inferior – he was on to something there. He was relatable. He connected with me. In doing the simplest things, he became a face and name that I would always remember. Knowing how valuable his time was, those precious few minutes that he gave to me were an unexpected gift. I felt love, from a virtual stranger. And again, there it was – joy.

There was no "moment" with Jhay that cemented his name and spirit within me. And I think that is the real point of this story. I am convinced that we all have an amazing ability to touch people's lives every day. And we don't know we have this ability. I think that was Jhay. He has no idea the extent to which he affected my life then and now. By the simple action of being authentically Jhay, he changed my life. He reminds me of who and what I want to be.

I WANT MY MOMMY

Given my requirement to know and understand everything that was happening to me at all times, I was not the easiest patient for doctors and nurses. It's not that I treated them badly. It's just that I wanted to be informed. I am a little bit of a control freak, I suppose, and that translated to me wanting to be in control of situations that, often, were not meant to be in my control. Nurses were almost always accommodating and walked me through whatever impasse we had reached. I simply wanted to understand what was happening before it happened.

After my thirteen-and-a-half-hour surgery in 2006, I started chemotherapy after that surgery. For five days, I had what is called intraperitoneal chemotherapy. During surgery, they placed two plastic tubes into my abdominal cavity, and instead of feeding chemotherapy drugs through the bloodstream, my chemotherapy drugs would be placed directly into my abdominal cavity. Each day, approximately one gallon of fluid was placed through these tubes into my abdomen to kill any cancer cells that might be attached to the organ tissues within my body. My particular cancer attached to the outside of tissues and was not contained within my bloodstream. This gallon of fluid was put in and left for twenty-three hours, at which time they would then drain whatever fluid was remaining, and I would have a one-hour reprieve until they filled me up for another twenty-three hours.

The process of infusing this large amount of fluid into my abdomen was not really painful, but I do remember that my swallowing became more difficult as the drugs entered my abdomen. I'm not a difficult patient, but, at times, my anxiety would get the best of me. Interestingly enough, the best solution to the problem was holding my mom's hand. There I was, a thirty-eight-year-old man who still needed his mother.

My mom rarely left my side while I was in the hospital. She would take breaks to go to the cafeteria or take a walk, but she slept in my hospital room every night for weeks. I was at the end of a one-hour reprieve when the nurse came in and said it was time to infuse another gallon of chemotherapy into my abdomen. She was ready, but since my mom was not present, I was not. I told her we had to wait. Most nurses I ever encountered were incredibly understanding. This one wasn't, and she told me that the infusion had to be done. With clarity, I remember yelling at this nurse, and, in fact, it is likely that I even cursed at her. She was not going to start my chemotherapy. I didn't often get angry, but at that moment, she was not listening to me, so I felt I had no choice.

In just moments, my mom returned, and the chemotherapy began. She held my hand, and I was safe. This moment is one that baffled me for a while because I really am an independent person. I live alone. I have climbed the corporate ladder. I own my own real estate company. But in that moment, I still wanted my mom. And it wasn't just that I wanted her there. In fact, every part of who I am needed to have her there to make everything okay. I'm not a parent, but I know what it means to need a parent. I felt joy, yet again. Joy, from my mother's hand.

Illustrated in all of these stories is the reality that joy can and does exist in the midst of some of the most grueling moments of life. Paying attention and focusing on the intention that you created before starting chemotherapy can have lasting effects on your experience with treatment. I believe that even though pain exists in the process of chemotherapy, joy can flourish and be more empowering than the pain. Hiding in the shadows of moments are pockets of joy that you will miss if you don't keep your heart and eyes open to the possibility that there is more to this experience. It may sound crazy, but I believe embracing your cancer diagnosis as a gift rather than a curse, will open doors that will allow you to embrace the reality of treatment and see things that you otherwise would never see absent your diagnosis. Remember that wishing away these moments means you miss so many golden nuggets of love, joy, and connection.

7

# FINDING JOY IN THE CHEMOTHERAPY JOURNEY

Fear and pain have a way of taking over almost all other emotions in a person. When faced with these two things, it's as if nothing else exists, and everything else seems to disappear. The tendency to give in to fear and pain can be overwhelming and will be one of the hardest challenges you will face on your chemotherapy journey. You can't erase the pain or the fear that accompanies not knowing what your future holds. That said, you can shift your focus and look around when in those moments. Choosing to look around you when faced with a challenging circumstance can dramatically shift your experience and, ultimately, the outcome of that moment. Your intention should guide you, and it should be the driving force in everything you do as you navigate fear and pain. When you succeed at this, painful moments will be transformed to life-changing moments, and it really is as simple as it seems. You get to decide what you see in each part of the journey. Reminding yourself that joy and pain exist together might be the thing that helps you shift your focus away from the pain and look more toward the joy that is already there.

## MOTHER FATHER GOD

It was August 2006, and I was back in the hospital, this time preparing for what was expected to be a thirteen- to fourteen-hour surgery, followed by up to six weeks of recovery in the hospital after surgery. I finished my first surgery and chemotherapy just over a year prior and, through a routine annual scan, had been diagnosed yet again with a recurrence of my appendiceal cancer. Prior to August, I visited my surgeon and oncologist, both in California, to get their opinions. Living in North Dakota now, I had to make some tough choices. Ultimately, I chose a surgeon near home and found a new oncologist who would treat me.

As I prepared for this major surgery and more chemotherapy, friends again showed up with their love and support. My friend, Carolyn, is a reminder of the joy and light that exists in all of us. She always seems to radiate joy. Carolyn wrote an amazing prayer for me. I printed it out as I wanted to read it before my surgery and then found I had forgotten to bring the prayer to the hospital. I remember telling my mom about the prayer and how disappointed I was that I had left it at home.

While living in California, my parents attended church with me at Unity of Berkeley. The service bore little resemblance to the liturgy-filled mornings of my childhood Lutheran congregation. It was a strange experience for them at first, as we paused for a five-minute meditation during each weekly service. I remember my dad telling me about all the things he thought about during that meditation period – he had to fix the shelf in my garage, he needed to replace the washer hoses, etcetera. By the end of their time with me, I really believe they had an understanding of the person I had become spiritually. This church service was so radically different than what they attended and far from the experience I had as a child. In the beginning, I think they were uncomfortable, but, ultimately, I believe they came to appreciate much of it. But truthfully, I was never completely sure.

Now, as I lay in a hospital bed, on the morning of this thirteen- to fourteen-hour surgery, I was surrounded by my family. My parents. My brother and his wife. My sister and her husband. Nieces. Nephews. It was an awkward moment as we waited for the hospital staff to come in and wheel me off to surgery. In these moments just before surgery, I hesitated about whether or not to communicate to my family what I wanted from them. I knew what I wanted but would my family think I was weird? Would it be uncomfortable? I decided to risk it.

I asked them all if they would do me a favor. I reminded them all how lucky they are to have someone to go to bed with each night. I told them the one thing I craved, more than anything, was the touch of another person. I asked them to never take for granted that leg on which they rest their foot while lying in bed at night. That touch is something that binds people together. I asked them all to gather around my bed, and I told them that, more than anything, I just wanted them to place their hands on me – anywhere on me. And they did. As I lay in that bed with my eyes closed, I felt hands on my legs, my chest, my arms, and my head. I felt love, and I felt connected to all of them.

In the silence of my hospital room, my mom prayed. She said, "Mother Father God ..." And that's all I remember. Because you see, in that moment, I knew my mom understood me. She prayed the way that we prayed at

Unity of Berkeley. In a moment, I felt not only the love of my mother but a new kind of respect from her. In life, I think many of us fail to recognize that it is the tiny things that you do or say that can have the greatest impact on those around you.

I went off to surgery with a sense of calm and peace, knowing that I was not only loved but supported in the beliefs I had formed as an adult. I no longer prayed to "Heavenly Father," as I did in my childhood church. But in that moment, my mom assured me it was okay. When they left California, I wasn't sure if they understood my church; now, I knew they did.

## THE SPA EXPERIENCE IN SURGICAL ICU

In September 2004, I went to surgery with the understanding that a laparoscopic procedure to remove my appendix would have minimal recovery time, and I would be back to work in a few days. Waking up and being informed that the laparoscopic procedure was abandoned because they found cancer around the appendix was not great news. Worse yet, was the long incision they had made in my abdomen. That incision was painful, and you don't realize how often abdominal muscles are used until they are split open with a knife and forced to heal. Sneezing was the worst. Even clearing your throat hurts.

Since I was unable to shower after this first surgery, a certified nursing assistant came to my room to give me a sponge bath. She was not a chatty person, and, to be frank, it was clear she did not like her job. The sponge bath that ensued is one of my worst memories of being diagnosed, initially. She needed to clean the incision site and did so without regard to the pain or discomfort I might endure. It was excruciating, to say the least. While it didn't last long, that painful moment always stuck with me, and I remember never wanting to go through that again.

Moving ahead to August 2006, I had just completed a thirteen-and-a-half-hour surgery. They administered hyperthermic intraperitoneal chemotherapy on the operating table and then sent me to the surgical intensive care unit to recover for a few days. My body had been forced to endure a long surgery and was now fighting to recuperate. As I lay on that bed in surgical intensive care, with a breathing tube down my throat, I was unable to talk or protest in any way. As I saw her walking toward me – a nursing assistant carrying a sponge and basin of water – I felt myself panic as I had flashbacks to that horrible experience a little more than a year prior.

Even in the midst of this panic, I imagined what life must be like for a quadriplegic who is dependent on others for care. What must it be like to be an older person living in a nursing care facility when you are unable to care for yourself? I was afraid for what was about to happen and yet still found myself grateful that this was a temporary situation for me. In the back of my mind, I just reminded myself that whatever pain there might be, it will be short-lived and temporary.

As she approached my bed, though, something strange happened. I felt a sense of peace and calm as she looked at me, smiled, and said she was going to wash my hair and clean me up a bit. It's difficult to explain, but the way she said it was almost as if she knew I was afraid. While my surgical incision was quite long after my first surgery, this one extended all the way from my pubic bone up to the rib cage, so it was even longer than before; essentially, they opened me up as much as they possibly could. For some reason, I was not afraid. When she touched me, it was similar to the experience I had when my family touched me prior to surgery in my hospital room.

Over the course of the next five minutes, I experienced the gift of love from a complete stranger as she washed my hair and cleaned my incision site. Careful in every move she made, it was clear she understood my situation and knew how vulnerable I was. That moment, after a grueling operation and a long recovery process pending, was one of the most joyful experiences of my life. I don't know her name. I wouldn't recognize her if I passed her on the street. Nevertheless, she is part of me. Looking for joy means it shows up, even in the surgical intensive care unit.

## IT FUCKING HURTS

After a thirteen-and-a-half-hour surgery, your body needs some time to recover, obviously. I woke up in surgical intensive care. While probably not completely true, I was in a room with tons of light, and the bed was in the middle of the floor and not against the wall. I had a central line in my neck for intravenous access as well as a urinary catheter. I had a bag attached to my abdomen, an ostomy (or poop bag), that would ultimately become permanent. I had a tube up my nose, which would be used to feed me in the coming days, and finally, I had a breathing tube down my throat that went into my lungs to keep me breathing. I opened my eyes and saw people but could not talk. It was the strangest feeling.

They asked me questions, and I wrote, with a pencil and paper, to answer them. While not always easy to read, they managed to comprehend what I was writing. I have come to believe, after being given pain medications many times, that these drugs not only inhibit pain receptors but they also inhibit other parts of us – mostly our brains, I suppose. I don't curse a lot though I'm certainly not an angel. My mom hates the 'f' word. She can tolerate almost any curse word – except an f-bomb. When asked by a family member how I was doing, I (inhibitions lowered) wrote out, "It fucking hurts." Even in the midst of seeing me with tubes coming out of all kinds of places where tubes ought not be, I managed to make them laugh. After such a long and difficult operation, my family managed to connect in joy over a simple statement. I'm fairly certain my mom smiled, too.

And, for the record, the following days proved that statement to be true. It really did hurt. But coming back to my intention for seeing joy, I have not recalled the pain in recent years, but the joy has most certainly remained.

## JUST A LITTLE SIGN LANGUAGE BETWEEN FRIENDS

I met Noelle on my first day of classes in college. I went to a private Christian college, and so, being the good boy that I was, I attended chapel at 10:00 a.m. on that first day. There were no classes scheduled at 10:00 a.m. so every student had the opportunity to attend chapel – daily. As I walked in, I saw this girl in the chapel. My memory has painted a picture of this traditional girl wearing some kind of lacy outfit. She was proper, almost. I'm not sure what struck me about her, but I sensed a friendliness as I sat down and said hello. We chatted, and, as it turned out, we both had the same class following chapel. That was the beginning of what would become the greatest friendship of my life. Noelle and I would go from being two naive kids from small towns to adults that cherish and love one another without condition. We traveled the country in a minivan, sleeping in the back for three weeks, seeing cities from New York to Maryland to Tennessee. I have never known friendship like the one I have with Noelle. In 2002, Noelle married Mike, and he defies every definition of friendship. I didn't believe it possible to love him as much as I love her, but, in fact, I do. In 2011, I had the great privilege of traveling to China with both of them to meet their daughter Emily. They are family to me, in the same way my parents and my siblings are family.

It was a couple days before my third surgery, a surgery that would be similar to my second one in that it would last approximately thirteen hours. I endured more chemotherapy on the operating table and possibly more after the surgery. It was different this time because I knew what was going to happen. After my second surgery, I endured a long path to recovery and was quoted many times saying, "I will never do this again." It wasn't easy. And yet here I was, preparing myself to check back in the hospital to do it all one more time.

The night before my surgery, we were all gathering at my sister's house to have one last meal. I pulled into the driveway at the same time as my mom and as I got out of my car, she asked me to get something out of the back seat of her car. Without much thought, I opened the back door and there she was – Noelle. As grateful as I was to Noelle for flying in to be with me for my surgery, I was equally grateful for Mike, her husband. The gift of their friendship is something I never take for granted.

I have said many times that I really believe the surgery is easier on the patient. I know it can't be easy for my parents, my friends, and family to endure hours of waiting outside an operating room in a hospital. Putting the life of your child, friend, or sibling in the hands of someone else for a thirteen-hour surgery is a heavy burden. After this long third surgery, I was again sent to the surgical intensive care unit. With a central line, a urinary catheter, a permanent ostomy, a tube up my nose for feeding, and a tube down my throat for breathing, I was ready to begin the recovery process one more time. With the tube down my throat, I was once again unable to talk. Of course, I wrote notes to people with pencil and paper, as I did before. Noelle has always had a special place in my life. As I lay there on the bed, beaten down by a grueling operation, Noelle and I signed back and forth. Years back, we had taken sign language together and there we were, connected in a way that reminded me how fortunate I was. Here it was again – joy. Joy in the simple act of sign language between friends. Joy existed in that painful moment because I chose to look.

## SOMETIMES NURSES KNOW MORE THAN DOCTORS

As I've said before, I really believe that nurses are the backbone of medical care and treatment. While physicians make the decisions and give the orders, nurses have a sensibility about them that goes beyond pure clinical diagnosis. Nurses almost always care for and, at the same time, provide love to their patients. They can't help it. It is, by nature, who they are.

I have had cancer three times. I have endured three surgeries and three hospital stays, along with chemotherapy on three different occasions. In all of that time, I can honestly say I never believed I would die. While a little crazy, it just wasn't what I saw for my life. Initially, I saw cancer as a mere obstacle to overcome, but ultimately, I would learn cancer was a gift that would teach me more about life and love and joy than I could ever learn – without the diagnosis. I learned to live in those moments of discomfort and pain. I would learn to see joy in those improbable moments.

In early December 2007, I was in the hospital recovering from my third surgery – the thirteen-hour long procedure which included removal of additional portions of my colon and small intestine, as well as more chemotherapy on the operating table. After waking from surgery, I was advised that they were unable to reverse my colostomy, so I would have to live with it permanently. I was tired. I had lost more weight, now weighing in just above 100 pounds.

My parents were right there with me, constantly insisting that I walk to ensure a speedier recovery. And, of course, I knew they were right, and I would eventually recover. After all, I had done this same thing just one year ago. Unfortunately, this hospital stay led to a post-operative infection, and pathologists worked diligently to find out what antibiotics to use; however, cultures take time to grow, and so I continued to get worse. At one point, my temperature had escalated above 104 degrees Fahrenheit. At that time, I remember, with absolute clarity, the confusion of the world around me. I remember being in a hospital bed surrounded by people, all talking and debating what they were going to do. It was as if I was in a foggy hazed world, and yet I could hear everything. The world around me was blurry, and I knew I was desperately ill. Of all the times I've been sick, this time felt different, and I was more helpless than I had ever been. In that moment, for the first time in all I'd been through, I just wanted to die.

In that moment, I was so exhausted and felt like I just couldn't take the pain anymore. I was incapable of making my own decisions, and my strength was gone. Being resigned to death, the next thing I can recall was something akin to a vision. Grandma Leila suddenly "appeared" in front of me. My maternal grandma had died five years earlier, in December 2002. It wasn't as if I saw a ghost-like vision of her floating above me. I didn't see her, and she didn't really talk to me. It was an odd experience, maybe more like a feeling than an actual vision. I recall having this overwhelming feeling that my grandma was present. Regardless of what it was, I felt that she was telling me that it was not my time to die, and she coaxed me into moving through the pain of this infection.

After I had this experience, I remember a physician at the foot of my bed. My parents and sister were also around my bed, along with a nurse who was asking for guidance from the physician on how to reduce my fever as we waited for pathology to determine the best course of antibiotic treatment needed to fight the infection. With the most cold-hearted response, I can still hear the physician asking the nurse a question. He said, "Have you given him Tylenol?" As the nurse responded that they had given ibuprofen, he advised her to try Tylenol and see what happens. He turned. He left the room.

Hopelessness is the feeling that best describes that moment for me, as the physician turned and walked away, but that feeling would be short-lived. As he left the room, the nurse took control of the situation. I was laying in the bed, sweating but having cold shivers at the same time. The nurse was on my left and as I turned to look up at her, she leaned down, placed both her hands on me, and got close to my left ear. She spoke to me words that will, for as long as I live, comfort, and sustain me. In a calm and almost whispered tone, she said, "Kipp, I know what we need to do. You're not going to like it. But I know what we need to do." This was my third time with cancer. I had never wanted to die. And in the one moment when death was my preferred choice, this nurse spoke to me with love, and provided wonderful joy. I had been committed to looking for joy, having been through this twice previously. I often wonder if that moment would have been memorialized to such an extent had I not been programmed to look for joy. Would I have seen it? Would I have heard it? Too often, people focus on the "loudest" feeling – that feeling of pain. In this moment, I believe I heard her because I was so intentional about my quest to look for joy. Always looking. And for the record, she knew exactly what to do. And it worked. And I didn't like it. She put ice under my armpits, between my legs and in every other part of my body that would hold an ice pack. It brought down my temperature and the infection subsided.

I don't know her name. I wouldn't know her face if she was sitting across from me (as is the case for so many others I've encountered). But she lives within me. Her spirit, her kindness, her gentle touch, and love live within me forever. I will never forget her kindness and love. And she doesn't know it.

## A BATTLE WITH THE CATHETER

Sometimes you just need to laugh – even if it is laughing at yourself. I don't recall this story from memory. I was told the details, after the fact, because I was either "happy" on pain meds or sleepwalking – or perhaps a combination of those two.

My mom usually stayed with me, in the hospital spending many nights in a really uncomfortable hospital chair. Occasionally, my dad would step in so Mom could go to the hotel, sleep in a real bed, and get a break. My dad is one of the kindest and most loving people I know. His approach, however, can sometimes appear a little rough around the edges, as he prefers getting to the point more quickly. He doesn't like to dance around whatever the issue is, and I've always liked that about him. Some people work so hard to avoid hurting feelings, it is often difficult to figure out what they are asking or saying. He just says what's on his mind and I think I've taken on that same quality from him now, as an adult.

It was the middle of the night. I awoke and told my dad that my hospital gown was wet and I needed a new one. He looked me over, and seeing a completely dry gown; he told me to go back to sleep. He went back to his chair and did the same but apparently, I was insistent on having a clean hospital gown because when dad woke the next time, I was heading away from my bed, apparently trying to go to the hallway to find a nurse. Given that my urinary catheter bag was attached to the bed, and I was trying to walk to the nurse's station, I was stuck in one place. Being tethered to the bed via a urinary catheter was preventing me from getting far.

At that point, he summoned the nurse, who got me a new gown, and I slept the rest of the night. I love this story because my dad got to tell it over and over. Parents hate to see their children suffer, and I can't fathom the agony my mom and dad went through as they watched me recuperate from each surgery. But having a moment like this provided amusement to everyone, and the image of me trying to get down the hall while a urinary catheter held me in place – that's funny. And silly. Joy, in the ridiculous.

### I THINK YOU NEED TO GO TO THE HOSPITAL

I had my third surgery on December 5, 2007, and I remember the day mostly because it is my niece, Darian's, birthday. I didn't want to hijack her birthday, but that was the day my surgeon wanted. It's hard to argue with a surgeon's schedule, and I wanted to have surgery early enough in December so I could be out of the hospital for Christmas. I was intent on not having Christmas in a hospital since I have young nieces and nephews, and being able to watch them open presents at home is what needed to happen. If I was in the hospital, I knew my entire family would also be there.

I struggled with a post-operative infection after this surgery and, as a result, lost quite a bit of weight. I was weak but my parents were always good about making me walk to build up my strength. Eating was difficult as it always led to extreme abdominal pain but this happened the previous year when I had the same surgery and so I knew it would eventually get better.

As I continued to slowly recover, I was finally able to leave the hospital several days before Christmas. I left the hospital with a urinary catheter but, at least, could be home in my own bed. I remember not feeling well and being incredibly weak, even lying on the bathroom floor after taking showers so that I wouldn't pass out. I hid all of this from my family because I just couldn't be the one to ruin Christmas. My family had given so much of their time, energy, and love during all my hospital stays; I couldn't bear the thought of taking away this holiday. But inside, I knew I was not doing well, and my recovery was moving backward instead of forward.

On Christmas Day, we all went to my sister's home. It was nice being around family and seeing the energy of the kids was healing in its own way. Even so, my body was not keeping up, as I was incredibly exhausted. Later in the evening, I asked if I could go upstairs and lay on my sister's bed for a while. My mom helped me to the bedroom and got me settled in and comfy. When I took off a hoody-style sweatshirt before climbing into bed, my mom saw me with my shirt off, and I could tell she was surprised at how skinny I had become. At the time, she didn't say anything, but I knew she was worried. I could sense she was holding back tears as she left me, having just seen how my body was wasting away.

Moments later, my sister, Tami, appeared at the door. My sister is a nurse, and at the time, she was working as a trauma nurse in the emergency room at the largest local hospital. She had been working in the ER for many years. As she stood in the door looking at me in the bed, her eyes filled with tears, and she said just one thing, "Kipp, I think you need to go to the hospital." Without hesitation, I replied, "I think you're right." Not only can I recall the love of my sister in that moment, but the love of a concerned mother. I have imagined the conversation that ensued as soon as Mom got back down to the living room. I know she left me in that bed with one mission. She needed to get me to the hospital. And she enlisted Tami to get it done.

As we checked in at the hospital emergency room, my weight was eighty-nine pounds. I was unable to stand, barely long enough for them to take a chest x-ray. More than the debilitation of that experience, though, is the comfort felt when a family comes together. Cancer can be an awful thing. But, at my lowest point ever, I was mindful of the awesome things happening all around me. My body was weak. But my soul and my spirit were strong – and joy-filled. Years later, I still remember the love and joy during those moments. I have put aside the pain, and how ravaged my body was. But joy remains.

If I have successfully conveyed anything through my stories, I want it to be that joy really does exist simultaneously with pain and fear. And while I know this to be true, I also know that the burden of seeing this lies within each person. You must have a willingness to overcome the distractions of pain and fear. Embracing the intention that you create to look beyond those hard moments will open up new memories that will not only change your experience of chemotherapy but your life. Using an example, let's see if I can help you understand what I mean. Consider that you have an itch on your nose. You know it itches, and you desperately want to itch it, but you also know you do have the ability to just sit with the feeling. Your brain is telling you to itch your nose, and yet you are able to continue doing something else while enduring the sensation. I know you've been in this situation where you couldn't itch because of whatever is preoccupying you in the moment. I believe pain is another sensation – just like the itch – and you do have the ability to recognize that pain while simultaneously looking around you to take note of the joy that may be happening at the same time. As I've noted, I firmly believe joy exists in parallel to pain, so reducing pain to the same category as an "itch" will, I believe, help you move into intention and feel, see, and experience moments as you've never done before.

# CHANGE YOUR LIFE EVEN AFTER CHEMO

Now that chemotherapy and treatment are over, many people think life can get back to "normal," and things will be better. In reality, the future likely means regular scans or tests to ensure the cancer has not returned. Or it may mean ongoing treatment to keep your cancer at bay. Whatever it is, the world will push you to return back to those moments prior to cancer. And while it is true that many things will be easier, I challenge you to continue embarking on that quest to find joy. In my experience, I have found that joy while doing chemotherapy was easier to spot because I was so focused on my health and getting better in those moments. The reality of life is such that you will be easily distracted, easily pulled in multiple directions by the obligations in your face. When life gets busy, and you get stressed or overworked, it might be simplest to return to that victim mentality. But choosing to continue with your mindset of intention even after you have finished treatment will be as rewarding in the future as it has been for your chemotherapy journey.

While I acknowledge it is sometimes hard to find it, joy

does exist even after treatment, so I challenge you to continue looking.

## CHEMO BRAIN: IT'S REAL

For those who have not heard the term "chemo brain" before, let me define it. Chemo brain is the transformed and mentally compromised brain of a person who is undergoing chemotherapy. Many chemotherapy patients experience an inability to focus and a decrease in the ability to retain and process information. As toxic drugs enter our bodies, they can and do affect virtually every aspect of our being. It is not unusual or uncommon that these drugs also affect brain cells. While many continue to function and go about their daily lives as before chemotherapy, many do not. I experienced this and found it nearly impossible to read, write or do anything that required me to think and process information while undergoing chemotherapy.

Playing cards was one thing I could do during my first cancer journey while living in California. Over the course of almost six months, my parents and I played cards. We spent countless nights sitting at my kitchen table playing Hollywood Rummy. My mom kept score and those moments around that table made the difficult process of recovering from chemotherapy much more tolerable. Though my energy was often low, we played. And we played. And we played.

What I did not realize was my mom was keeping score of all those games in the same notebook. Hollywood Rummy requires scoring a seven-round game. After seven rounds, the person with the lowest score wins, and my mom had circled the name of each game's winner throughout this notebook. Shortly before my parents left

California to go home to North Dakota, my mom sat down to tally up who the overall winner was. It felt similar to some kind of tournament. We had played all the games; now, it was time to announce the champion, so to speak.

So, who won? Surprisingly, all three of us tied. Hundreds of games played and, in the end, each of us had won the same number of games. We all laughed and thought it was a curious coincidence. What my parents don't know is that, for me, that coincidence was symbolic of something bigger that happened, in all our lives. For six months, I lived with my parents as an adult. I realized that not many grown children have an opportunity to really get to know their parents, as adults. We got to know each other. And that silly little game, with the score tied, showed me that we are all equals. My parents know me and how I've changed. And I, too, had an opportunity to see them. We became friends and were no longer simply parent and child. Through a simple game of cards, we became connected in a new way. Crazy joy.

## TEA WITH ANN GARAT

I often wonder: What makes a moment a "moment?" What is it about those particular times in our lives that are captured, almost like photographs, and instilled to memory – instilled in such a way that it can be almost instantaneously recalled and remembered, at any point in the future. I'm not sure I know the answer. My life is filled with moments that would, to the average person, seem inconsequential. But they aren't. The simplest and tiniest gesture can change the course of someone's life. The things you do and the things you say have the ability to touch people's lives – in ways you can't even imagine.

In 2005, Ann Garat and I were both undergoing

chemotherapy in Berkeley, California. We sat next to each other during several chemo sessions, and I got to know her. I didn't know her well, but we were partners in a venture – chemotherapy. She was older. She had kids and grandkids. She talked about them, a lot. When we finished our treatment, life took over and we didn't see each other much. Shortly after I finished chemotherapy in 2005, I quit my job and moved back to North Dakota. Ann and I stayed in touch by exchanging occasional emails.

In Winter 2006, I got in my car and drove around the country for six weeks. I visited friends along the way, making a special stop at Ann's loft, in Emeryville, California. Ann was doing okay but she was back on chemotherapy and didn't have the energy to meet up for lunch or dinner. In truth, there was nothing out of the ordinary about this visit. Just me visiting a friend at her home.

Ann lived in a unique warehouse space that had been converted to loft condos. In fact, I had looked at a space in this building when I was home shopping several years earlier. I loved the space, and I have a vivid recollection of sitting in this big comfy chair just under a massive window. She sat next to me, served tea, and provided amazing conversation. I adored this woman and felt incredibly blessed to have met her. I remember thinking how she and I would be great friends if I still lived in the Bay Area.

After a couple of hours of conversation, I left. My road trip was nearing the end, so I would soon head back to North Dakota. After several months passed by and life returned to normal, an email showed up in my inbox one day from Ann's daughter. She informed me that Ann had passed away. Receiving this email was a blessing. I never met her daughter, and yet she knew enough to send me an email. Even though Ann had died, receiving an email from her daughter meant that Ann spoke of me. It was a reminder that I touched her life.

While it may seem crazy, I still think of Ann Garat whenever I drink hot tea.

A MOTHER KNOWS EVERYTHING

It was May 2005, and I finally finished six months of chemotherapy. I was still not able to eat, having been fed intravenously for the previous five months. I would continue receiving nutrition through my port for a while, but I was done with chemotherapy. I had been planning a party in my head for quite some time. When the end was reached, I wanted to have an "I Survived Chemo Party" at my house. While it would be a time to party and celebrate my completion of treatment, it would also be a party to thank my parents. They would get a chance to meet friends, and it would be a sort of "going away" party for them, as they would soon return to North Dakota. I invited my friends and Mom, of course, prepared delicious food. It felt like the beginning of my normal life again as my energy was high, and being surrounded by friends was incredibly joyful.

During my six months of chemotherapy treatment, I managed to maintain a positive attitude, for the most part. Having had the benefit of my epiphany in Spain, I was constantly on the lookout for something good, even in the darkest moments. I usually found something good in most bad situations. In the interest of full disclosure, however, I will admit that I had moments where I felt beaten and destroyed. I felt sadness, and I felt loneliness. In those rare moments, I wanted to do the simple things. I wanted to eat food again (I was tired of being fed through a port in my chest), I wanted to ride my mountain bike, I wanted to run,

I wanted to work. I felt angry and needed to vent my frustration. Because of the port in my chest and the fact that it was accessed all the time for my TPN feedings, I was not able to easily shower. During those five months, I resorted to baths.

Since my parents knew I took baths, I would take some time, when down, to cry in the bathtub. I couldn't possibly burden my parents with anything else. They were already watching their child go through chemotherapy. They had to eat, while I sat and watched, being fed through a tube to my chest. They had given up so much. And I was so lucky and fortunate, it seemed unthinkable for me to ask them for support when I was feeling depressed. I would take a bath. And I would cry. Then, I felt better. And nobody knew.

At my party, I was hanging out just taking in the energy of the room. I was standing alone, watching friends connect through conversation. From a corner nearby, I saw my mom talking to a friend of mine. As I eavesdropped, I heard my mom say, "Kipp used to go in the bathroom and cry, sometimes. He needed to do that; I think. He doesn't know that I know." I walked away, smiling. Joy.

My mom has always been connected to me. And in that moment, I remember feeling such gratitude and joy. She knew that I needed alone time. She knew that I didn't want to be consoled. She knew that I needed to appear strong, even though I wasn't at times. It was so good to feel respect from my mom. I had just finished chemotherapy, and what was showing up in my life still? – Joy.

## I'LL GET A TATTOO NEXT YEAR

In order to understand this story, you need to know a little about my mom. In her entire life, she never smoked and never drank alcohol. She got drunk one time at a Jaycees convention – but that was an accident, and she didn't even know she was drunk until the bed started spinning, and she asked my dad to take her to the hospital. My dad had to explain "bed spins." I would never say my mom is naive. She is smart, self-assured, and independent. In general, she is someone who "plays by the rules" and doesn't get too far outside the proverbial "box."

When I was younger, I would have never considered getting a tattoo. This would have been unthinkable, but the world has changed, and the rules have relaxed a little. My brother and sister also have tattoos. My mom didn't always understand the tattoos but loves us all, nonetheless. After my mom's fifty-ninth birthday, she told us she was going to get a tattoo when she turned sixty. I loved that my mom was going to do this, as it was something that most people would never expect from her.

After telling us about her plans, we had brief conversations throughout that year about what she would get and where. She really wasn't sure. But the anticipation made for good conversation. As we approached August 2006 (her birthday month), I was diagnosed with cancer for the second time. With the distraction of more tests and a lot of research to figure out what my next step should be, the thought of Mom getting a tattoo sort of took the back seat. I scheduled surgery for the first part of August and was told I would be in the hospital for three to six weeks following surgery. We celebrated her sixtieth birthday in my hospital room, and, of course, she thought about nothing but me getting better. I, however, remember thinking that she was supposed to be getting a tattoo that day.

We celebrated, and I don't recall even discussing the tattoo, but it was on my mind that entire day. Eventually, I was released from the hospital, and Mom was there for every step of my recovery. Life would eventually return to normal, and the talk of a tattoo faded.

As her sixty-first birthday approached, we reminded her about the idea she had for her sixtieth birthday. I think my sister, Tami, made the appointment and we paid for her first (and still, only) tattoo. I can still see her sitting in that tattoo shop cringing, as the sound of the needle gun started up. She was tense but did great. Her tattoo incorporated a treble clef with a butterfly – this was perfect since music has been such a guiding force in her life. I know she loves it.

While that sixty-first birthday may have seemed like a simple thing – getting a tattoo – it was far more to me. As I watched my mom get that tattoo, all the memories of her sacrificing for me flashed through my head. This amazing, incredible, unconditional-loving person was doing something really outside her comfort zone. She probably learned that from her dad – my Grandpa Leroy. He taught us all something similar. Life changes. People change. But at the end of the day, family is always constant. Sharing this moment with my mom brought such joy to me.

BETTY

The power you have to touch another person's life is incredible. Every day, you walk in the world with more power than you can comprehend. What strikes me more than this is the fact that most people don't acknowledge or even know they have this power.

Betty was the cleaning lady where I worked, and she usually had a Swiffer in her hand as she wandered around the office at night. I worked at Keller Williams Realty, at the time, as a licensed real estate agent. I've never been a morning person, so I often worked late, and consequently, my hours would coincide with the cleaning crew. Betty was a talker, and I remember having moments when I thought to myself, "Oh no, here comes Betty. I have work to do." But that was only in the beginning. Through our many hours of conversation over the years, she taught me to slow down and be present in the moment, and she reminded me that family is most important. Even though I was taught this by my parents, diving into work and focusing on career goals meant I needed a little reminder. She worked with her daughter and grandson, and she understood that connecting with other people is one of the most important things you can do while living on this planet. She taught me about loving strangers.

What's interesting about all the things I learned from her is that she never spoke about any of these things. She taught me by simply being Betty. Over the course of a couple of years, I forged a friendship with her. While we never saw each other outside work, and I never knew her last name, she was a part of my life – a person with whom I connected. She made me a better person.

I never told Betty how much her friendship meant to me. She died in 2014. I hope she knew we were friends, and I hope she knew what respect I had for her. It may sound crazy to some, but Betty still lives within me. I think of her often, especially when I'm using my Swiffer to dust. Silly, perhaps, but she touched my life. I really don't think she knew. Joy.

## NEWFOUND RESPECT FROM CHILDHOOD

Throughout my childhood, I recall weekends at the lake. I grew up in North Dakota, and during the summer, my family would go to our cabin at Lake Metigoshe nearly every weekend. We did everything from water skiing to sailing, but my dad never bought us a jet ski. That is, to this day, a sort of running joke. We were fortunate and blessed, my parents working hard to provide us with more than what we needed. We had fun, but my dad hated jet skis – so, of course, we wanted one.

My dad worked long hours. I always feel compelled to add that my mom also worked, though her work was the more difficult job of maintaining a house filled with three children. She did everything. We were all lucky. My mom was home nearly every day when I would arrive from school, and my dad was not home much. These are my early memories of how it was. I also recall, however, that each and every summer Friday, my dad would arrive home sometime mid-afternoon, and we would pack the Suburban and head to the lake. Even our dog, Mitzi, paced the floor when Dad arrived home. It was a tradition, and it seemed to happen year after year, weekend after summer weekend, like clockwork. That was my childhood.

In 2014, my sister and I, now adults, bought a small lake place together. The memories we had from childhood were so amazing that we wanted to share that experience with Tami's kids. Now, as when I was a child, I would work diligently to get home on Friday afternoons, grab my dogs, and head to the lake.

One Friday in the summer of 2015, I was wrapped up in some project at work. I wanted to get to the lake before my sister and parents, so I had plans to leave the office early. It never happened. I became engrossed in my work, and when I finally was able to leave, I was irritated with myself and my work which led to me being cranky and irritable. By this time, everyone else had arrived at the lake, and I had been receiving text messages asking about my arrival time. Ultimately, they ended up eating dinner without me, which only made me more upset – not at them, but at myself.

After packing my bags, I headed out the door with my two dogs, and we got in the car for the short forty-five-minute drive. For whatever reason, driving always seems to calm me. There is something really liberating about driving down an open road. More liberating is winding down a two-lane highway in beautiful lakes country. I was starting to relax, and as my mind wandered, I thought about all those times we did this when I was younger. I have two dogs and my duffle bag. I thought about how difficult it must have been for my mom. She was responsible for three small children, food for the entire weekend, clothing for all of us, and more. We never once thought about how much work it was to travel every weekend to a cabin with three little kids, a dog, and a husband. I felt gratitude and love. Grateful for a mom who worked so hard for three little kids that took everything for granted.

Smiling now about how fortunate I felt, my mood was better. I still couldn't let go of how incompetent I felt. A smart leader would have better control over his time. If I really was good at managing my company, it would be easy to leave. And yet, here I was, hours late. Then it hit me. My dad did this every weekend when I was a child. In that moment of realization, an actual feeling of joy came over me. Wow. My dad had far more responsibility than I do. He owned a farm implement business – a business that relied on four months of the year for probably 90 percent of the income for the year. Farmers worked in the summer, and this was his busiest time of the year. How was he able to leave the office every Friday afternoon?

By the time I arrived at the lake that day, I had developed a sense of tremendous respect for my dad. On that short drive, I realized what he did all those years ago. And I realized how difficult it was, having just experienced it myself. He may not have been home every night when I went to bed, but he made sacrifices every weekend to be with his family. He always knew what was important – and he still does. That day, I became even closer to my dad, which I would have thought was impossible.

A stress-filled day turned joyful, seeing for the first-time memories of a father's gift. He gave us his time – and it took me years to realize how valuable that gift was. I believe that keeping my mind open to the intention of finding joy is why I was able to have this realization.

## IT REALLY IS ABOUT THE LITTLE THINGS

Friendship is a funny thing. Is it possible to be friends with someone you have only met on one occasion? Is it possible to consider someone a friend when you don't even speak to them on a regular basis. My answer to both is an unequivocal yes. In fact, I believe you can have a strong friendship in this situation.

Mayland was a United State Postal Service employee. The year was 1998, and I was traveling the country – each week in a different city – installing new computer systems in post offices. After installation, I would train the postal employees how to use the new software. It was a fun year, but the travel got tiresome – real fast. Often, people think corporate travel is exciting, but the truth is, after a long day of work, all I wanted to do was eat and relax. And working on my own, it got lonely at times. In addition to this, I was away from my dog and my home for nearly every week of the year.

I was working in Collegeville, Pennsylvania on, this particular occasion – a bedroom community just north of Philadelphia. It was a typical week of installing and training. Then, after a long day, Mayland asked me if I would be interested in a home-cooked meal. The truth is, I was tired and really wanted to go to my room and be lazy. But Mayland was so interesting. From the moment I met her, I remember an energy of love and kindness. That was, mostly, not the vibe I got from employees who were being forced to learn something new. I accepted her invite and ventured to her home for dinner that night.

As I arrived at her home, she looked at me and asked, "What should we have for dinner?" Being someone who doesn't cook, I could not help with that question. She said, "Let's go to the garden. We'll figure it out." As we walked through her garden, she picked a little of this and a little of that. I remember her picking lots of squash, a vegetable that doesn't get me too excited. We went back to the kitchen, and she began cooking up our dinner, which included inordinate amounts of squash. We had an amazing meal and even better conversation. I learned that Mayland is a Quaker. I had never met a Quaker. I learned that she loved men's college gymnastics – her passion for this sport was intoxicating. I learned that she has a solid commitment to the 42nd "Rainbow" Division (her husband's army unit in WWII), attending their reunions around the country each year. I left her home that night with a feeling that is hard to describe. It was, most simply, the feeling of connection. After only one evening, I knew this woman loved me. And I loved her. We connected, over a shared meal, as strangers, but I left her home that night, knowing I had a new friend for life.

The years would pass quickly, and Mayland and I never spoke, over the telephone or otherwise. We would send and receive annual holiday letters but never spoke. One year, I remember writing about her in my letter; and as it happened, she also wrote about me that same year. Our letters crossed in the mail, and we each received them, simultaneously reading the story about the other. We really were connected. We are connected.

In the past several years, we talked on the phone more often. Interestingly, we both acknowledged wanting to call throughout the years, but both were never sure how to initiate such a call. Our relationship had become close but was defined by the infrequent connections via postal mail. Now, when we do speak on the phone, it is rarely for less than an hour – usually more. In one conversation, I talked about this book and how I was frustrated with myself because I was not getting it done. We all have a tendency to beat ourselves up, I think. I was disappointed in myself and really felt like the book needed to be completed. In her simple way, she reminded me that it wasn't the right time for me to finish. She has a way of trusting that everything will happen when it should, a Quaker belief. The guilt and disappointment I felt was not self-serving; she encouraged me to let it go. That ability to accept people as they are is part of her DNA. Now, the other thing I love about her is that she won't allow bad grammar. She's a smart, intelligent, kind, and loving person.

Every year I receive a holiday letter from Mayland, and she always includes a note along with the typed holiday letter. One particular year, she wrote about my book and provided guidance and suggestions on how to move forward. It is crazy how she has this ability to push you a little bit while at the same time assuring you that the speed at which you move is perfect. She is a part of who I am today.

In August 2016, nearly twenty years after meeting Mayland, I drove through Pennsylvania on a road trip with my ten-year-old nephew, Jaxx. We parked our RV in her driveway for the night, and I had an opportunity not only to reconnect with her but also a chance for Jaxx to see what an amazing person she is.

Mayland continues to remind me of the importance to pay attention. If I wasn't paying attention so many years ago, imagine what I would have missed. A friendship that has spanned years. A friendship that is strong. A friendship that is meaningful. To this day and forever, I am connected to Mayland. Joy – because I said yes to a dinner invite. And now, joy each and every time I eat squash. Mayland and squash are synonymous for me.

KITTY

When I think of Kitty, my first thoughts are: smart, independent, gorgeous, determined, self-assured, beautiful hair, great dresser. I have known Kitty for as long as I can remember. She was married to my great uncle, Bill, who passed away when I was just a child. Even though I don't remember much about Bill, I remember going to see him at work one day. We walked in the front door of the bank, turned right, and there was his desk – sitting back in this corner. He gave me a lollipop from his desk drawer, and that's my memory of Uncle Bill.

Kitty and Bill had two small children when he passed away. I don't ever remember seeing her sad. Of course, I was only a kid, so I'm certain she had moments of sadness – who doesn't? For some reason, Kitty has always been part of who I am. I really don't know how to explain it.

When I was just a little boy, I took her a rose bowl on Valentine's Day. Honestly, I don't remember why or how this started. She was special to me then; she is still special to me now.

My mom worked extremely hard. I could never deny that fact. My Grandma Leila also worked hard. My mom and her mom both worked in the home – they were full-time moms. That's all I ever knew. Kitty, however, owned Kitty's Fashions on the square in downtown Kenmare. She was a different kind of woman. In the eyes of a pre-adolescent child in the 1970s, I noticed her because of the differences. In a way, I have always idolized her. She is strong in ways that most people aren't. She has this determination about her that appears innate – as if it's easy and normal. In a way, it's not fair – I remember being on a pedestal in the eyes of others, and I don't recommend it. The fall is rough.

Kitty will never fall off the metaphorical pedestal I've erected in my mind. I still receive letters and cards from her. Although I think of her often, Kitty doesn't know because I don't take the time to write back as often as I should. She knows I love her, and I suspect she knows that we share some kind of special connection. But she can't possibly know how she has influenced my life. Mostly because I've never told her.

It was a typical Tuesday. I was with my Mahjong ladies – Dianne, Kerri, and my mom, Billiette – at Dianne's house. Every Tuesday, I play Mahjong with three great ladies, all of whom I adore. At any rate, we were taking the usual break to have cake or something, and Dianne told a story. She was talking about her son, Michael. She recalled how Michael told her about this lady, Kitty, who was nice to him. He used to sit on the sidewalk and draw in the dirt with a stick. And he remembered Kitty – the lady who was nice to him.

I always knew she was special. In that moment, I wondered how many other people knew? And did she? We all have an amazing ability to touch and change people's lives every day.

FRED

Fred Shulak is a man who probably doesn't understand the impact he had on my life in a moment when I was struggling internally. Our paths crossed for only a brief time in August 2009. Honestly, I could tell countless stories like this one because, it really is the smallest of things that make big impacts.

In August 2006, I had my second surgery – a thirteen-and-a-half-hour surgery that was supposed to leave me with what was sold to me as a "temporary" solution to help my body heal. I would leave this surgery with an ostomy that would be reversed and removed after one year. For those that don't know, an ostomy is when they cut a hole in your abdomen and divert your colon or small intestine to this opening, where a bag is then attached to collect any waste. In short, and more crudely, it means I now poop in a bag. As stated, it was supposed to be temporary.

However, when I had a third cancer recurrence in 2007, I underwent another thirteen-hour surgery, and they were, in the end, unable to reconnect my colon to the rectum. With the cancer recurrence and the extensive scar tissue, my surgeon felt like it would never be possible. In the first year of having an ostomy, I didn't stop living. I biked from Vienna to Budapest with friends in Europe and continued my other activities without restrictions. But honestly, I never really embraced the idea of having an ostomy as I knew it was temporary. I had some issues but just muddled my way through, knowing that it would soon be corrected. After my third surgery, when they couldn't reverse the ostomy, I decided it was time to embrace this "poop bag" and figure out how best to manage my life and this new appliance.

In August 2009, the United Ostomy Association of America was having its bi-annual convention. They only have a convention every two years, so I decided to road trip it to New Orleans, with my friend, Chad. We had a great road trip driving from Fargo, North Dakota to New Orleans, Louisiana. I have great memories of that trip.

While attending the convention, I met Fred in the exhibit hall. I am not good in large groups. It's one of the things that just makes me nervous. One-on-one, I am a relaxed conversationalist and can be quite interesting, but groups are not my thing. Being amongst so many people and not knowing anyone, I was starting to feel overwhelmed. Fred befriended me, and I felt comfortable in the group because of him. After meeting Fred, I opened up and explored the different booths that were set up in the exhibit hall. When Fred asked me to dinner that night, I was surprised. He and his group of friends have been meeting for years at these conventions, and he included Chad and me. I am certain that it was, to Fred, just another dinner with friends. To me, it was a reminder of how easy it is to touch other people's lives. The memory of that simple dinner with new friends at a convention is something that brought great joy to me at a time when I was trying to deal with my new reality of "pooping in a bag."

## LET'S MEET AT STARBUCKS

Sometimes in life, it's the simplest moments that can have the greatest impact on our lives. I have learned, over the years, how to find joy in really challenging, troubling, and improbable moments. And while that's all well and good, I have noticed that it is often easy to skirt the joy found in the obvious, everyday moments.

It was May 2015, and I had been in San Francisco for almost two weeks, helping my friend Rob as he recovered from hip replacement surgery. I stuck close to his home for most of the time, as he had some ups and downs with the recovery process. Toward the end of my stay, I ventured to the East Bay, where I lived from 2001 through 2005. My friend, Carolyn, picked me up at the BART train station, and we headed off to lunch.

We ate at a tiny little hole-in-the-wall cafe that most people in Oakland love – Mama's Royal Cafe; the cafe is just a block from where I used to live. We walked past my old house and then headed to Starbucks to sit and chat. We sat outside at the coffee shop, which was overlooking a gorgeous water retention pond. Houses sat atop what appeared to be a mountainous wall, and the homes literally butted up to the edge of this cliff. The scenery was lovely, and the weather was perfect. We sat there for hours and just chatted. She is someone with whom I connected strongly years ago. And when you have that kind of connection, it doesn't really matter where you are or what you're doing. When the moments of togetherness are few and far between, they tend to be memorable.

On that gorgeous day in Oakland, I found this pool of joy that has stayed with me. It was just a simple, ordinary meeting between friends. But it reminded me how to define the meaning of true friendship. Continuing to look for joy after chemotherapy is not always easy, but finding it requires you to hold your intention to look. Paying attention on this day means that I can see joy in the simplest things that happen in daily life.

## SANTA CLAUS

I met Duane in April 2013. He owned his home in a small town north of Fargo. He really did look like Santa Claus; I guess that's why almost everyone in this small town called him Santa. Over the course of a year, I got to know Duane. He was a great reminder, to me, about judging a book by its cover. While he may have looked like Santa and had the charm and flair of Santa, he was so much more – so I never called him Santa. He was Duane to me.

I'm not sure anyone would argue with me if I said Duane probably wasn't the best father. In conversations with him, I came to realize that he knew he made mistakes. In fact, those mistakes seemed to haunt him as he wanted desperately to repair the broken relationship with his son, but could not find the courage to take that first step. Over and over, I tried to get him to make that first move. At the end of the day, he just couldn't.

What keeps us stuck in the past, I wondered. Duane grieved for the loss of his wife, and he grieved because diabetes left him with neuropathy in his fingers, which prevented him from playing guitar – something he loved. I remember telling him about an iPad app that resembled a guitar. I told him that, even though he would not be holding a guitar in the traditional sense, he could still create music in a new way. He had no interest. He just seemed to focus on what he had lost.

In my mind, I really wanted him to take a bold leap forward and create this new life, absent his loving wife and absent his ability to play guitar. For a long time, I felt like I was not being successful. Then I realized, I had an agenda that was counter to his. I didn't live in his shoes and couldn't know or understand why he was unable to make the decisions that, in my view, could have had a profound effect on the course of his life. Duane died a little over a year after I met him.

When his son, Shawn, called to tell me that Duane had passed away, I felt deep sadness. That sadness was for the loss of someone who had become a real part of my life. I didn't talk to Duane often, but I thought of him regularly. He imprinted his "self" into my life, and now, knowing he didn't get to fulfill some of the things I knew he wanted; I felt sad for him – and for those whose lives could have been changed.

There would be no funeral for Duane. Shawn invited me to the family service, a gesture for which I was grateful. I had only known Duane for a little over a year. I was the real estate agent trying to convince him to sell his house and move on to better things. The truth is he wanted to sell. He desperately wanted to move to Las Vegas and reconnect with his son and get to know his grandkids. But he was so afraid. How had I become so entangled in his life? And yet, there I was feeling gratitude for that entanglement. While I was unable to attend the family service because of another commitment, the gesture made by his son, is something I will always remember.

I believe there are many people in that small town who think they knew "Santa" – and maybe a few did know him. My suspicion, however, is they knew what he showed on the surface. He was jolly and quite a lot of fun. I know that he loved his son and had a desire to bond with grandchildren that knew little about him. He wanted that more than anything. I remember him saying it over and over. And yet, it didn't happen.

For me, Duane is a reminder to always live in the possibility of what might be. Live without fear. Many knew him as Santa. To me, he will always be Duane. But I will admit, whenever I see a Santa Claus, Duane is right there, too. I smile. I feel joy. I feel gratitude, having known a man that loved his family, but was unable to tell them – or show them.

ROAD RAGE

My office is in a prime shopping location in Fargo, North Dakota. The building has a Starbucks, as well as other shops, offices and eating establishments. That said, our parking lot can get full and there are always moving cars. In the spring of each year, the owners of the building allow the construction of a temporary greenhouse in the front parking lot. This brings in more cars and closes off the typical traffic flow.

One day during the spring season, I was leaving my office. As I approached the greenhouse, I had to veer outside of my lane to go around the greenhouse. As I did this, a lady coming from the opposite direction gave me the nastiest, dirtiest look possible. I was livid and, in my anger, responded with a hand gesture that was not polite. She scowled at me as if I had done the worst thing possible.

As I continued on, I let my anger swell. There was plenty of room for her to move over. Couldn't she see that I had no choice because of the greenhouse placed in the parking lot? I found myself now agitated and driving aggressively. Such rudeness on her part was disappointing. And then, for whatever reason, my anger, in an instant, just dissipated. Almost at that moment, a realization came over me: we all have an amazing ability to touch people's lives every day, and we don't know it. I say this all the time and believe it to be true. In that moment, a rude lady changed my day. Why was I allowing this? I realized that I, too, could make a choice. My anger did not serve me, and it certainly did not serve anyone else. I let it go. I decided to give the driver the benefit of the doubt – perhaps she did not see the greenhouse. Perhaps she was having a bad day.

I can't say that I'm always able to do this. The world is full of confrontation and moments that cause us to respond in less than loving and joyful ways. I get it. But for whatever reason, that moment stands out. And it continues to stand out, whenever I encounter situations beyond my control. I have cut off my fair share of people on the road. Many of those situations were inadvertent as I simply did not see the car coming.

As I move through the world now, this moment continues to "take front and center stage." I am ashamed of how I reacted and use this as an example to do better moving forward. I also use it as a reminder that I also have the ability to affect other people's lives with my actions. It may seem a little crazy, but I now find myself looking for something good and something joyful in those irritating moments behind the wheel. I'm not perfect. But the bitchy lady in my parking lot made me a better person in her small little way.

## LISA ROHM VISIT

In high school, I was involved in Luther League, a church organization for young people. Every four years, a national youth conference would be held somewhere in the country. In the summer of 1985, that youth conference was held in Denver, Colorado. We spent years raising money to attend this conference and when the time came, we chartered a bus and filled it with young kids from North Dakota. I recall horrible, awful memories of the trip to Denver as our pastor coordinated a stop at a western-themed bible camp along the way, and so we spent the night sleeping on the ground in teepees. I can still remember looking up at the hole in the top, just wishing the night would pass and we could move on to our next stop. We still laugh about how awful that night was.

When we arrived in Denver, our accommodations were nicer, and the trip started getting better. There were thousands of young people from all over the country in attendance, and I vividly remember our gathering at some monstrous venue in Denver. We filled a huge arena, and it was truly a great experience as a kid. However, what I remember most about that trip was this red-headed girl who wandered the halls of the hotel, chatting up anyone who would listen. She was self-assured, outspoken, and confident. In my youth, I was none of those things. Over the course of those few days, I got to know Lisa Rohm. When the convention came to a close, we exchanged mailing addresses and, over the course of the next several years, maintained a connection via letter writing – a lost art these days. Back then, that was the only option. Phone calls were expensive, and there was no such thing as the internet or email.

The next time I saw Lisa, I was graduating college. That was 1991. As adulthood brought on responsibilities and career became the focus, Lisa and I lost touch. But she was still a part of me. In fact, I can, to this day, tell you her mailing address from memory. I was only seventeen, but Lisa was an example of someone I aspired to be.

In February 2015, I drove from North Dakota to Iowa, so I could be present with my best friend as she and her husband embarked on the home buying experience. They were having a home inspection done, and so I decided to be there with them. I wanted to see the house, and I am also a licensed real estate agent. Coincidentally, Lisa lives in the same metropolitan area, so I decided to shoot her an email and see if she might be up for coffee.

It had been nearly twenty-four years since I last saw Lisa. We sat and talked and connected, just as we did so long ago. What I found fascinating about that visit was the fact that our connection was even stronger than it was before. We have both grown and matured. We met for a short time as children, and yet, we held tight to what we shared, and today, I have an amazing friendship that has spanned more than thirty-five years. Distance may separate us, but our hearts and souls are connected, and I still need Lisa.

It was just a typical Saturday morning coffee appointment, but it was an experience of joy in my everyday life – a joy that was built from a simple chance meeting between two kids who needed each other so many years ago. And I still need Lisa.

THE BIKE PICTURE

Sometimes, it's really the simplest things that make us smile. My nephew, Jaxx, was eight years old and assigned, by his teacher, to write a story about a photograph. The photo was a bike. I never saw the photo. I only saw the story he wrote:

> The Bike picture reminds me of my uncle Kipps story. My Gma told me in Mexico. He was riding his Bike and somthing was harting. I don't remieber the rest But he had cancer 3 times that not alot or people suvred with it but he did 3 times. IT IS SOOOO COOOOl!!! and he still loves to Bike!!!!
>
> Written By: Jaxx  5-6-14  May 6", 2014
> To: Kipp Harris

When my mom shared this with me, the feeling of joy was overwhelming. How simple. And so, what? He wrote a story. But if you dig deeper, this is about a kid paying attention to the way we live our lives. I was encouraged by the fact that he saw his uncle living passionately after enduring pain and discomfort over and over. Through my life and my story, he has an example to follow in his future. We are all products of our environment. To know that my journey had such a positive influence on a kid was incredible. We forget the extent to which kids listen. They hear everything and knowing that he took something good from my long cancer journey means that I did something right. Joy – in every day, little, tiny moments.

Recognizing the power, you have to create joy not only for your life but for those around you can be a great influence as you navigate life after chemotherapy. Personal tragedy can serve as a wake-up call allowing you to see the joy that exists in the world. Gaining new perspective during your treatment can mean that life after cancer is better than ever. I hope my examples of moments where I saw joy after chemo can serve to inspire you to continue on the mission to be intentional.

# CONCLUSION: PAIN AND JOY EXIST SIMULTANEOUSLY

One thing I know beyond a shadow of a doubt is that joy and pain exist simultaneously in the same moment. Your inability to see and feel joy is only a result of your unwillingness to look for it. Authenticity breeds love, joy, and connection with other human beings, and I believe there is nothing else that you need to survive on this spinning planet we call home. Gregory Todd Jones started an organization called "Living Wide," and they subscribe to the motto: "We may lose control over the length of our lives, but we never lose control of the width." In short, he believed in his final years that it didn't matter the length of his life, but rather, it was the width that mattered.

When you open up to the possibility of intention and choose to seek out joy, you will find it. My hope is the stories of where this worked for me might help you to start on your journey. I know it has changed my life because I am now more willing to open up and share my experiences with others. My pain is not a burden to anyone but rather a gift to be shared with everyone. As humans, most of us want to help others – don't deny others the opportunity to help you.

Any journey with cancer is a difficult one. Knowing that fear and pain will be a consistent theme throughout the experience can be a hard reality for many people to face. If you follow the advice I've given in this book, I believe you will not only find joy in the cancer experience, but you will learn how to look at all of life's challenges in a new and positive way.

## STOP LOOKING OUTSIDE YOURSELF

Sitting on a beach, writing in my journal, I came to an epiphany that changed my life. I decided to find joy in chemotherapy. What started as a simple idea to "bear" the burden of chemotherapy turned into a way of life for me. My life has been forever transformed as the most mundane things find me looking for something good. There is good everywhere – I know. And I know because I look.

And I look because I listened to my inner self. Listen to your inner self. Look inside and hear what your soul is telling you. Stop looking outside yourself for answers about who you are. Sometimes, the hardest thing to do is open up and be vulnerable, but if you do this, I guarantee your life will change in ways you can't imagine. Being honest with your feelings and reaching out to friends and family for support and love is not you being weak – it is you acknowledging the fact that your diagnosis affects more than just you.

## INTENTION IS THE KEY

Looking for joy in improbable places is not easy. When you are in the midst of an experience that is painful, your mind tends to focus on the fact that you are not happy. Or you focus on the negative reaction to whatever might be happening. Because of intention, I have been able to change my focus, in the midst of some uncomfortable moments.

I'm not telling you that life won't be hard. I'm not telling you that life won't hurt and be full of painful and uncomfortable moments. Frankly speaking, that's life. But if you have to experience those things – and we all have to – then why not try to shift your focus. Make an intention to look for joy. Regarding pain as a sensation similar to an "itch" can be the impetus for moving through it and seeing other things in that moment. It really is that simple.

I know there are pessimists who say that not everyone can do this. I don't believe them. You have choices. You can choose to focus on the nasty, horrible, awful experience, or you can look around and just take a chance that there might possibly be something joyful in that same space. I've done this – and I've shared the stories here – and it changed the course of my life. At my lowest weight, I was eighty-nine pounds, and I still remember the X-ray technician who helped me stand so she could quickly get a chest x-ray. I could barely support my own weight because I was so weak – and yet, I have to think to recall how awful I felt. In a flash, I can remember the technician who cared for me. That's joy. And that's simple.

Intention is the key. You must decide that you want to look.

CANCER ISN'T A FIGHT

I acknowledge that this is a hard sell for many because we live in a world where cancer is constantly talked about as this evil, horrible thing. Loved ones retort the message that society has embraced – fight cancer. And yet, here I am saying the opposite, "Stop fighting cancer."

For me, it makes much more sense to find a way to live during the course of your treatment. Entering a fight for six months of chemotherapy and recuperation time just didn't work for me. I didn't want to look back on my time during chemotherapy and view it as something that "interrupted my life." It was my life. For whatever reason, I got cancer. It seemed logical that I should embrace that and move forward, paying attention to all the love and joy that was present along the way.

What I found to be the most interesting after completing my first six months of chemotherapy: I was happier at the chemo clinic than I was at my job. Having spent a good amount of time analyzing that craziness, I now realize that life, in its "normal" state, is full of distractions and obligations. When you're being treated for cancer, you become much more myopic in your focus. The little things that used to bother me just didn't matter anymore. The focus of my energy was on getting well. For me, that was living with cancer – and, in my own way, ensuring that it exited my body so I could move forward with my life.

The distinction is small, but important. I believe it is a change in focus. You already have cancer, so fighting just seems counterproductive to me. Your time and energy, in my opinion, can better be utilized by focusing on the life you currently have. In the end, if cancer is what takes your life, living to the end would seem more meaningful than fighting to the end. I get it. Life is valuable and amazing. But at the end of the day, you have zero control over what happens. You can move through the treatment and hope the odds are in your favor. You can pray. But ultimately, fighting just doesn't help, in my opinion.

We have been fighting a war on drugs for years – and yet, is drug use down? It also seems as if there is this odd perception that if you don't fight, you are giving up and simply accepting death. Nonsense. Live with cancer. Embrace it. Honestly, cancer was a gift that changed my life. I believe that more people could benefit from the joys of cancer if they stopped fighting. In fact, there is research suggesting that the mere fighting mentality contributes to less-than-ideal outcomes when treating cancer patients. Nothing you do will eliminate the fear and pain you have during the process of cancer treatment, but I can tell you, from my experiences shared in the stories here, that I remember the joy I saw because of my intention. I don't remember or focus on the pain and fear I had in those moments.

## MOMENTS MATTER

*"We do not remember days, we remember moments."*

— CESARE PAVESE

This book is really about moments. It's about average, ordinary people seizing opportunities to make themselves great without the help or guidance from anyone else. We're all amazing. We can all teach each other but we don't always have to be taught. Today's eagerness to capture insight has created an economy of self-help seminars, life coaches, and retreats. These all have value, but this book is not about me teaching you – it's about you teaching yourself. It's about reminding you to look inside yourself for the most important lessons of all.

If you become intentional and start looking for joy, I

can virtually guarantee you will see things and find joy you never knew existed. The stories in this book are living examples of that idea.

## MY BIGGEST LESSON LEARNED

I used to think my job as a corporate, regional manager didn't matter. I studied math and chemistry in college and wondered how those pursuits would ultimately change the world. At heart, I'm a do-gooder, and for a long time, I believed I "should have been" a social worker or nurse or physician – those are people that really make a difference. What I've come to understand is that you, without hesitation, have an incredible ability to touch and change people's lives every single day. I know I said this in the book, but it bears repeating in this last section.

If you have finished the book, you know of countless stories where seemingly unmemorable moments took place. Most of the moments chronicled here touched *my* life, and I am mostly unaware of whether the other person involved has any recollection. This proves one thing to me: If other people can have such an impact on my own life, is it not possible that I might also impact others? And perhaps I don't know it. And perhaps you don't either.

I hope that after reading this book, you will understand that creating an intention to seek out joy can and will have an impact on your life and the lives of others. Most notably, it will distract from the realities of the fear and pain associated with chemotherapy and cancer treatment in such a way that your life will be better for having gone through treatment. While this may sound like a nonsensical position to take, I am proof (having endured cancer and chemotherapy three times) that this can be and is, in fact, the case. I am a better person because of cancer.

My family is closer and more connected because of what we endured together.

What I now understand is that no job or purpose is meaningless. We all have an amazing ability to touch and change people's lives every single day, no matter what we do. Living a purposeful and authentic life with passion can and will touch the lives of others.

# ACKNOWLEDGMENTS

In the acknowledgments section of one of her books, Jodee Bock noted that most people only read this section to find out if they were mentioned. I always thought that was funny so I will first thank Jodee not only for our continued friendship but for her tireless work in reviewing my original manuscript for this book several years ago. She gave harsh critique when so many others were just telling me how brilliant I was; for that, I'm grateful and I believe it led to fine-tuning this book in ways that benefit the reader.

While I have dedicated this book to my parents, I must also acknowledge them here for their countless support over the years as I worked on this manuscript. Their continued love and support was unfaltering and none of this would be possible without their love and support. My sister, Tami, along with her family, has also been incredibly supportive over the years as she continued to support my ambitions. My brother, Todd, in his own way, has contributed to this work by just being someone that loves me. While he and I often see the world through quite different "lenses," we connect in love and his support has always been obvious to me.

I tell a story about Mayland Crosson in this book but it can't be said enough the extent to which her encouragement manifested this book. When my spirits were low and I was beating myself up for procrastinating, she would simply remind me that it wasn't time for it to be complete.

Mayland and I have only been physically together on two occasions but our friendship is one that has blessed my life in ways I can't recount here. I never believed in soulmates until I met her!

I met Noelle Andrew in 1986 on my first day of college and that day is still imprinted to memory as if it happened just yesterday. The memories we have created over a lifetime are some of my most cherished and knowing that her husband, Mike, and daughter, Emily, are now also my family is a blessing I will forever cherish. She exemplifies a kind of love and acceptance that makes this world a better place.

Dawn Omdahl brings joy to my world in ways that I simply can't convey in words. We travel together, laugh together, poke fun at others together, and have inside jokes that connect us in ways that make my life meaningful and complete. She understands my mission in publishing this book and has supported and loved me through moments when things got tough. I'm connected to Dawn and can't imagine being here without her.

My buddy, J.L. Cleland, deserves special recognition because without him, I'm not sure I would have had the original epiphany that led to the creation of this book. His friendship over the years has been an example of someone really living life. He values relationships and experiences above material things and my connection to him is a surprise that life threw my way. I will forever cherish and value the many late-night conversations had by the massive stone fireplace in his farm house outside Topeka. Drinking wine and solving the world's problems together has sustained me in times when life seemed a little tough!

My dear friend, Carolyn Honey, is a constant source of love and light in the world and will forever be the one I call when I need to connect to something bigger than myself. She has a way of reminding me that we are all very small and there is something bigger that connects us all. She makes me feel loved and supported no matter the circumstance.

Dick Duey was someone that scared me; and in the end, he became one of the people I loved most in this world. Our political differences were substantial but they did not prevent us from being friends. Because of Dick, I now consider his wife, Anne, a dear friend who loves me and supports me. Anne has never stopped asking about this book and has continued to remind me that the world needs to hear this message.

I met Nancy Johnson in 1996 when I moved to Minneapolis for a job. Working together, we both "climbed the corporate ladder" and managed to stay connected through the years even when distance separated us. I don't recall a time during conversations with Nancy when she has not asked me about this book. Her continued and persistent support sustains me and leaves me with a sense of pure gratitude.

Sometimes (as noted in this book) people don't even realize the extent to which they impact another person. To that end, I will simply say the following people have loved and supported this book even though they may not know it: Elizabeth Porter, a girl I met on YouTube so many years ago; Patty Splawn, a former co-worker who inspired me in a recent phone call; Lisa King, a friend who reminded me that sunrises are important.

David Santilli and Wayne Church are two friends that provided me with an opportunity more than five years ago to begin the process of writing this book. Their generosity gave me the time and space I needed to begin this process.

Finally, I want to thank and acknowledge all the people who are subjects of stories in this book. Life is about connecting and their willingness to allow me to be a part of their story and their life is why this book exists.

# ABOUT THE AUTHOR

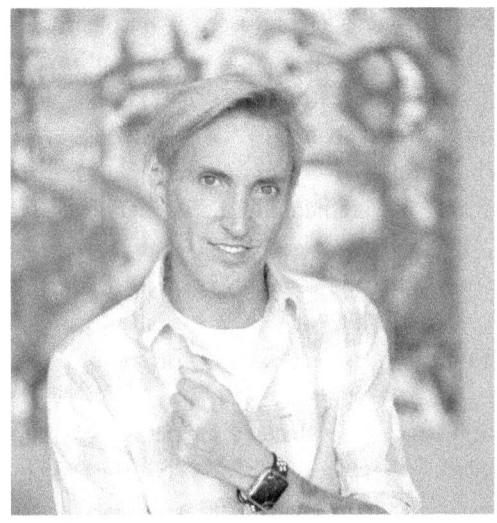

Kipp Harris is a real estate agent and speaker who spends his time working to make sure people understand that joy exists in really unexpected places. After college, he found himself working at a pharmacy software company. After working his way up the corporate ladder from trainer to sales rep to regional manager, he moved to California where he oversaw operations at three regional offices on the West Coast for an east coast-based company. He was happy and content, with a beautiful home, friends, and lots to do and see in the Bay Area. Additionally, he managed to travel and see the world and discover the diversity which had seemed lacking in his small hometown.

In 2004, after a day of mountain biking in Northern California, he suddenly ended up in an emergency room and later a post-surgical hospital bed only to get news of his first cancer diagnosis. That moment — and the years that would follow — are the well-spring of his book.

Since 2004, Kipp has endured three surgeries, three successive bouts of chemotherapy and three surprising journeys with cancer. His message is simple. Joy occurs in the most unexpected places, if you are intentional and look for it. He also believes that every person has an amazing ability to touch and change lives every single day.

This book tells the stories of the simplest moments that are captured and cemented in his memory because he chose to be intentional. His hope and message is not to instruct but rather aid others to look inside themselves to discover the inner gift that already exists. We all have what we need within ourselves and, too often, look outside for answers.

Having lived many places, Kipp returned, in late 2005, to the place where he started – North Dakota. Being cancer-free since December 2007, he now understands that life is really only about three things: love, joy, and connection!

To book Kipp as a speaker for your event, information is available on his website: ImprobableJoy.com

www.ingramcontent.com/pod-product-compliance
Lightning Source LLC
Chambersburg PA
CBHW050004230526
45465CB00003BB/1254